THE WORLD OF THE SENSES
AND THE WORLD OF THE SPIRIT

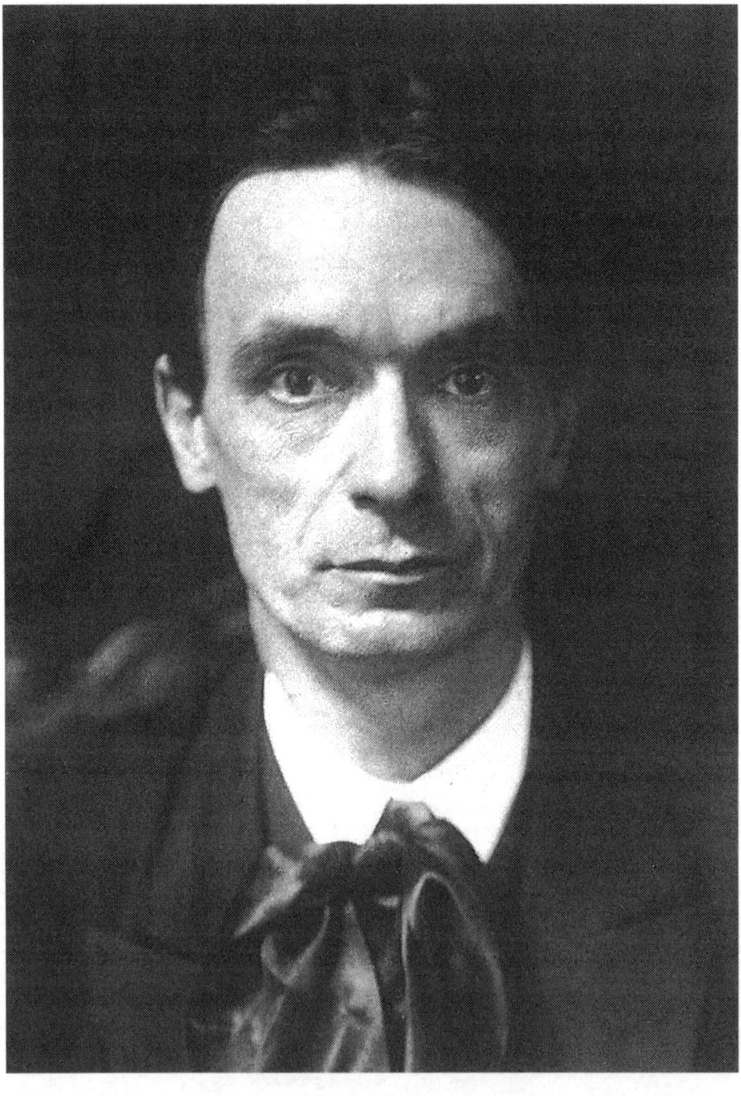

THE WORLD OF THE SENSES AND THE WORLD OF THE SPIRIT

Six lectures given in Hanover between 27 December 1911 and 1 January 1912

TRANSLATED BY JOHANNA COLLIS

INTRODUCTION BY MARGARET JONAS

RUDOLF STEINER

RUDOLF STEINER PRESS

CW 134

The publishers gratefully acknowledge the generous funding of this publication by the estate of Dr Eva Frommer MD (1927–2004) and the Anthroposophical Society in Great Britain

Rudolf Steiner Press
Hillside House, The Square
Forest Row, RH18 5ES

www.rudolfsteinerpress.com

Published by Rudolf Steiner Press 2014

Originally published in German under the title *Die Welt der Sinne und die Welt des Geistes* (volume 134 in the *Rudolf Steiner Gesamtausgabe* or Collected Works) by Rudolf Steiner Verlag, Dornach. Based on shorthand transcripts not reviewed by the speaker, and edited by Hans Erhard Lauer. This authorized translation is based on the latest available edition (1990)

Published by permission of the Rudolf Steiner Nachlassverwaltung, Dornach

A catalogue record for this book is available from the British Library

ISBN 978 1 85584 396 7

Cover by Mary Giddens
Typeset by DP Photosetting, Neath, West Glamorgan
Printed and bound in the UK by 4edge Limited

CONTENTS

EDITOR'S PREFACE

These lectures were given to members of the Theosophical Society in Hanover during the Christmas season of 1911. Rudolf Steiner's visit to Hanover and the programme of events had been announced in the 'Notice to Members of the German Section of the Theosophical Society', XII, November 1911, and in a separate invitation (see page facsimile on p. 92 with translation opposite). Rudolf Steiner formulated the title. The lecture on 26 December was preceded by the Section's Christmas celebration. The lecture on this date is also included in GA 127 (not presently translated as a complete course in English). In the New Year celebration on 1 January 1912, Rudolf Steiner spoke about the Dream Song of Olaf Åsteson. This talk is included in GA 158 (also not presently translated into English). The celebrations in Hanover ended on 2 January with a further lecture by Rudolf Steiner of which only notes remain.

INTRODUCTION

These lectures took place when Rudolf Steiner was still lecturing within the German Section of the Theosophical Society, and they were given to those members in Hanover. However, the term 'theosophy' has been altered to 'anthroposophy', following Steiner's later suggestion. A certain background understanding of theosophy/anthroposophy was thus assumed by him. The lectures have been carefully translated in accordance with a later German edition, rather than the previous English version.

One of Rudolf Steiner's fundamental objectives in all his activity was to endeavour to show in what way the spiritual world could be said to connect to and penetrate the material world, and thus avoid the traditional separating off of physical and spiritual (or religious) manifestation. He also knew too well how easy it is for a materialistic science to claim to have refuted the findings of anthroposophy; so, rather than disregarding the senses and the impressions they give to us—as might be in the case of developing a purely meditative path—his intention was to arrive at a greater understanding and enhancement of their functioning. It would then be by developing the power of thinking as a tool which could penetrate through and beyond them. The best exposition of this thinking capacity is found in his book *The Philosophy of Freedom.*

Steiner was later to explore the human senses more fully, describing twelve and thus going beyond the customary five. In these lectures he is dealing with the sense world as a whole, rather than specific ones, but he does give some unexpected insights into the senses of sight and hearing in particular. We learn for instance how it is that we experience colour. Spiritually, the senses reveal the world of the will, which is also an aspect of our physical bodies—it requires effort on our part to understand will as both a spiritual and a physical phenomenon.

The Gnostic teachers of the second century AD, to whom he alludes in the first lecture, commonly described the material world as having been created by a god less good and powerful than the highest divine being, a lesser creator which some identified with Yahweh of the Old Testament—but others even perceived it as the work of evil entities. Rudolf Steiner does not go this far, but he indicates that the spiritual divine beings had very different intentions for the formation of physical human beings. The adversary powers, however, especially Lucifer, interfered in the divine plan and the result was a more materialized human being. These descriptions must have come as quite startling when first heard.

We learn the different ways in which the physical, etheric, astral bodies and ego can be connected and the effects of the preponderance of one over the other, from which certain medical conclusions can be drawn. Disorder has been brought into these connections. Now we gain a better understanding of our glandular secretions, and how we have become beings who need to eat and digest—which would not have been the case had Lucifer not intervened. Steiner realized this would disappoint any gourmets in his audience! His listeners were also presented with the difficult concept of how to understand spirit actually becoming something material. What is matter or substance? Can we grasp the idea that spirit bursting into emptiness produces mineral substance? His explanation is carefully built up. Mysteries of space and time and evolutionary processes are also discussed, and how the human being is part of the cosmic whole and relates to the Spirits of Form—the Elohim for instance—a connection which in turn is made with the human ego and the blood. Steiner leads on to the astonishing idea that the human being of the distant future will be able to transform his senses and his organs in a mysterious way, in particular the larynx—which will have a certain reproductive power. The doleful future of a humanity which does not want to know about these things, and refuses to develop a higher consciousness, is brought before us.

But whatever the nature and origins of the senses, the way we should respond to our sensory impressions is to remember to receive the world around us in a mood of amazement and reverence and allow it to speak to us. This is far more important than we realize. To meet it with fixed concepts will, moreover, hinder our judgements; likewise states of excessive sympathy and antipathy. As Goethe before him showed, phenomena of any kind must first be received in a mood of quiet acceptance before drawing any conclusions. Premature concepts, judgements and opinions simply erect a wall and obstruct, leading to untrue ideas and confusion. Developing the right mood is a moral act and essential for really being able to receive what the senses bring to us. *This* is the truly scientific mode, not the dogmatic one so prevalent today.

In this period Steiner was also presenting a modern form of Rosicrucianism—a development of the attempt during the Renaissance by its founder, Christian Rosenkreutz, to unite science with belief, and in some respects these lectures are more challenging than others given around this time, such as *From Jesus to Christ* or *Wonders of the World*, which deal with religious and mythological themes. But only by trying to grapple with these difficult concepts can we really further the understanding of spiritual knowledge—not just as ideas or beliefs but also as a *science.*

Margaret Jonas, May 2014

LECTURE 1

HANOVER, 27 DECEMBER 1911

IN this cycle of lectures it will be my task to build a bridge between more or less everyday things, between experiences we might encounter in ordinary life and the most lofty affairs of humanity. This may show us one of those paths which lead on from our everyday life towards what anthroposophy or spiritual science can mean for our soul and spirit. We know, if we enter ever more deeply into what it is able to give us, that anthroposophy will flow into our feelings, into our will, and into the powers we need in order to come to grips with the many and varied events of life. And we also know, through the way we can experience the influences which are just now approaching us from the higher worlds, that anthroposophy is in some measure needed by today's humanity. We know that within a relatively brief period of time humanity would lose all certainty, all confidence, all inner quietness, all the tranquillity we need for life, if the revelations we describe as anthroposophy were unable to reach humanity in our present age. We also know that through this spiritual stream of anthroposophy two tendencies of people's thinking and feeling are approaching one another with some violence.

One of these is the tendency of thinking and feeling which has been in preparation for many centuries and has already taken hold of humanity everywhere in the widest circles, or will most certainly do so very soon. This is what we term the materialistic tendency of thinking and feeling; it is materialistic in the widest sense. And it is, as it were, clashing violently with the other way of thinking, the way which comes through anthroposophy and is the spiritual tendency. The conflict of these two tendencies, of these two ways of thinking and feeling, will become ever more noticeable in the near future. In the way it manifests we shall not always know whether we are dealing with a tendency of thinking and feeling which is undisguised in its materialistic presentation or which is, perhaps, another tendency hiding behind some mask or other. This is because there will be plenty of materialistic tendencies which will disguise themselves as something spiritual, and it will sometimes be difficult to see where materialism is hiding and where a spiritual tendency is truly to be found. In two lectures I gave recently I endeavoured to demonstrate in various ways how difficult it is to make the necessary distinction in this regard. In the first instance I tried to give a sense of how certain thoughts and ideas which can easily dominate us at the present time can make of us perfectly honest and upright opponents of spiritual science. 'How to refute spiritual science' is what I tried to demonstrate in the first of those lectures, which was then followed by another describing 'how to defend spiritual science' or 'how to substantiate spiritual science'.[1]

It was not my intention in those lectures to demonstrate everything possible in either direction. My purpose was to provide a sense of how numerous exceedingly plausible ways can be found by means of which the world view of spiritual science can be refuted. Nevertheless, those who cannot help but pour forth such antagonism from their soul should certainly not in every case be counted nowadays among the most dishonest individuals, for they are often in fact the most honest among those wrestling to find the truth. I shall not here present you once again with all the reasons which can be stated in opposition to spiritual science. But I must point out that today's habits of thought and ways of looking at the world do provide very well-founded reasons on the basis of which spiritual science can be thoroughly refuted. If we wish to refute spiritual science, if we want to seek out all possible reasons that can be set against spiritual science, we must ask the question: How can we reach the most thorough, the most fundamental refutation? You see, a person may acknowledge spiritual science from the very bottom of his soul, and yet if he then also familiarizes himself with the essentially materialistic ideas put forward by the sciences he will find it perfectly possible to refute spiritual science very thoroughly. To do this he must first bring about within himself a certain state of soul. This state of soul in a person who wishes to refute spiritual science involves adopting a completely and utterly intellectualistic point of view. What is meant by this will become clear when we view the matter from the opposite standpoint once we have grasped what I have here presented as my own personal experience. If we are familiar with the results of today's science while relying solely on our intellect, we shall find it possible to refute spiritual science very thoroughly.

But now let us pause while we endeavour to approach our task from an entirely different angle. You see, we human beings are able to view the world from two sides. One view arises when we, let's say, witness a beautiful sunrise where the sun emerges from the golden-red morning sky as though giving birth to itself and then spreads its brilliance across the earth while we immerse ourselves in the thought of how the sun's warmth magically brings forth life from the earth's depths in the ever-recurring round of the seasons. Or, when we observe the going down of the sun as the red sky at night grows dim until total blackness holds sway in which myriads of stars shine out, then we can become absorbed in the wonders of the starry sky at night. This view of nature all around us can fill us with the most profound delight. Such a perception resembles one of Goethe's fundamental ideas. He once expressed it so beautifully: As we look up to the wonders of the starry heavens and watch the circulation of the universe in all its glory, then surely we have a sense of how all these marvels surrounding us in creation only grow meaningful when they are mirrored in the astounded soul of a human being.[2]

We do indeed play with the idea that just as the air around us forms our being, just as it enters into us when we breathe and through the process it undergoes within us then builds us up, that just as we are an outcome of this air and its laws and its composition so are we in some way an outcome of the whole wide world which surrounds us with all that flows into us through our senses—not only in what we see but also in what we take in through the world of sound and all the other worlds flowing into us through our senses. The fact that we stand there before the external world of the senses and are an outcome of all those senses flowing together, and are able to tell ourselves that we have within us everything we perceive around us through all our senses, this fact enables us to understand that the meaning of all this is best fulfilled through the crystallizing out of the marvel which is the human being.

How truly are we then overcome by the notion expressed with such primeval passion by the Greek poet: 'Of all that is mighty in the world, the most mighty is the human being!'[3] How one-sided do each of the world's external phenomena appear to us! Yet in the human being all these phenomena seem to merge together into a one-ness when we view the world of the senses outside ourselves and then see the human being in its midst as a sensual being into which all else is flowing. The more closely we investigate the world, the more does the human being emerge before us as a confluence of all the one-sided phenomena of the universe. A thought enters into our soul when we cultivate within ourselves this feeling of the great wide world and the way it unites to flow into the human being, a thought filled with profoundly inspiring feelings: the concept of the divinely intended human being who emerges as though the deeds of gods and godly purposes had built up an entire universe whence they everywhere caused influences to flow which in the end combined in the most estimable of works then placed by those gods into the universe, namely the human being—an opus of the divine will!

This is how it was expressed by one who was contemplating the world of the senses with regard to the human being: In relation to the miracle of the human ear all of us are the music maker's instruments as are we also in relation to that other musical instrument, the miracle of the human larynx![4] We can marvel at much that is in the world; not to marvel at the human being who stands there in its midst is possible only if we are unfamiliar with the wonders of his configuration. But when in soul we immerse ourselves in such contemplations, then the thought arises: How great are the deeds of those divine spiritual beings who have brought this human being into existence!

This is one angle to be gained from a world view. But there is also another angle. This other angle is revealed to us when we develop a sense for the grandeur and potency of what we term moral ideals, when we look into our own soul and are struck by the significance of moral ideals for the world. A many-sided healthy human nature is called for if we are to sense fully how sublime are the moral ideals of humanity. In contemplating these moral ideals we can develop in ourselves something which may work within our soul just as powerfully as the wonders and revelations of the universe work on us from the outside. This comes about when we kindle all possible love and enthusiasm in relation to the moral ideals and aims of humanity. It may fill us with immeasurable warmth.

And then this sense of the moral ideals is joined as of necessity by the idea of the aforementioned world view related to the revelation of the universe through the human being. Those who have the strongest sense of the might of those moral ideals will also be most powerfully affected by that other thought and say: O man, as you stand here today, how distant are you from the lofty moral ideals which can blossom within your heart! How small are you in all your capabilities over against the greatness of the moral ideals which you might set yourself!

Only when our soul begins to grow can we assess its inadequacy over against those moral ideals. And the thought then dawns in our soul which helps us endeavour with courage and conviction to make the moral ideals a little more strong within us than they were before. Or else it can happen in some temperaments that the sense of inadequacy of the moral ideals begins to take root in the soul which then feels utterly shattered and alienated from the gods for the very reason that it does in fact have a strong understanding of the divinely willed aspect of the *external* human being's place in the world of the senses. Here I stand, such individuals might say to themselves, with everything I possess externally. Regarding yourself from the outside you cannot help saying: Yes, I am a confluence of the whole divinely created world; I am a being desired by the gods with a countenance resembling the divine! But then you look into yourself and there you see the ideals which the gods have inscribed into your heart and which are intended by them to be powers you can use. So then you feel the experience of your inadequacy gushing forth from your soul.

We have within us these two possibilities for looking at the world. Either we can regard ourselves from outside and be profoundly glad about our divinely desired nature. Or we can regard ourselves from within and be profoundly disappointed about our soul in its estrangement from the divine. With a sound sense of the situation we are bound to say: The forces which have brought forth the human being like a mighty extract of the whole universe are the very same forces which have also brought forth the moral ideals that are inscribed into our hearts.

Why is the one so very different from the other? This surely is the great riddle of human existence. In truth, neither anthroposophy nor philosophy would ever have come about in the world if the dichotomy just described had not arisen in human souls either more consciously in the realm of thinking or less consciously in the realm of feeling. The experience of it is the source of all human questioning and investigation. What has come between the divinely willed human being and the human being who is estranged from the divine? This is the most fundamental question of all philosophy. However varied the formulations and characterizations of this question may have become, nevertheless it underlies all human thinking and all human pondering. How may we gain an idea of how to build a bridge between the indubitably inspiring view of the external human being and the undoubtedly conflicting view of the soul leading to so much doubt?

The path that must be trodden by the human soul in order to rise up in a right and dignified manner to the highest questions of existence will have to be described in more detail. This will then tell us where the errors originate. In the world outside, in so far as it is dominated by external science, people will always say: Yes indeed, knowledge and truth will be the result if one has made the correct judgements. In order to characterize the fundamental error inherent in this presumption, that knowledge and truth will arise out of correct judgements, I recently employed a very simple comparison which I would now like to repeat here to show you that what is right does not necessarily lead to what is real.

There was once a small village boy whose parents always sent him to buy fresh rolls. They would give him ten pennies and he would return with six rolls. One roll cost two pennies, and for ten pennies the boy returned with six rolls. The little lad was not much good at sums, so he didn't bother to work out why he always brought six rolls home with him even though one roll cost two pennies. But then a kind of foster brother came to live with the family. He was more or less the same age, but better at arithmetic. He noticed that the lad was given ten pennies for the baker and he also knew that one roll cost two pennies. So he said: You should bring five rolls home with you. He was good at arithmetic and thought quite rightly that if one roll cost two pennies, then ten pennies would buy five rolls. And yet the lad came home with six. So the boy who was good at sums said: It's not right; if one roll costs two pennies and you are sent to the baker with ten pennies then, since two goes into ten five times, you can't possibly come back with six rolls. Someone must have made a mistake, or else you pinched a roll. And yet next morning the boy again returned home with six rolls for ten pennies. This was because in that village it was the custom that someone buying five rolls for ten pennies was always given six. It was a very agreeable custom for the people who needed only five rolls for their household.

Well, the boy who was good at sums was quite right; there was no mistake in his thinking, and yet his correct thinking did not agree with the reality. We have to admit that his correct thinking did not conform to reality for the very reason that reality does not always comply with correct thinking. You see, as in this instance, however conscientious and intricate the thought may be, which leads to however logical and correct a conclusion, the result when measured against reality can be completely and utterly wrong. This is always possible. Therefore a proof gained by means of thinking will never, but never, accord in any way with reality.

It is also possible to be mistaken in other ways with regard to the peculiar interrelationship of cause and effect when applied to the outside world. I will give you an example of this, too. Imagine a person walking along beside a large stream. Watching him from a distance you see him suddenly fall over the edge into the water, and rush to save him, but when you pull him out he is dead. So now you have a corpse. Perhaps, mustering all your ability to think logically, you will reason that he has drowned. Maybe there was a stone at the spot where it happened, so he stumbled over it, fell into the water and drowned. The sequence of thoughts is perfectly correct: someone walks along a river bank, stumbles over a stone, falls into the water and is dead when he is pulled out; so he has drowned. This is the only explanation. But with this particular individual it may not be the explanation. If we don't allow ourselves to be ruled by the links between cause and effect we may discover that at the moment when he fell into the river the man had a heart attack which caused him to fall into the water. He was already dead when he fell and only seemed to react in the way one normally reacts when falling into water alive.

So you see that in this case it is wrong to string together the external events of stumbling, falling into the water and drowning. It does not conform to reality because the individual fell into the water on account of being dead, and was not pulled out dead on account of having fallen. Judgements as wrong as this one about causes and effects, and much more subtle ones as well, are made all over the place in our scientific literature, but they remain unnoticed just as would have been the case if we had not investigated the matter of the man with the heart attack. All I am suggesting is that in fact, with regard to reality, our thinking is utterly incompetent; it is inconclusive and no judge of what is actually true.

So how are we to extricate ourselves from the morass of doubt and not-knowing if we can indeed not rely on our thinking being a reliable guide? When one has had experience in such matters and has concerned oneself a great deal with thinking as such, then one knows that it is possible to prove anything and contradict anything, so one is no longer impressed by the astuteness of philosophy. One can admire astuteness, but to rely on conclusions arrived at on the basis of the reasoning faculty alone is not possible because one knows that equally cogent conclusions proving the opposite can also be arrived at through reasoning. This is true of all things which can be either proven or refuted. Very interesting observations, especially those based on real life, can often be made in relation to this. There is a certain allure—though only a theoretical allure—in making the acquaintance of people who have reached a specific point in their soul development, namely the point where they sense and experience inwardly that everything can be proven or refuted, but who have not yet acquired what one might term a spiritual world view.

In recent weeks I have often been occupied with such thoughts in remembrance of a man I once met who possessed to a most remarkable degree a constellation of soul of this kind and who was thus unable to press on to a true comprehension of reality through spiritual knowledge. What he had attained was the realization that basically every philosophical statement could be either denied or confirmed. He was a professor at the University of Vienna, a highly intelligent man who died a few weeks ago, Laurenz Müllner.[5] This highly intelligent man was able to put forward with the utmost clarity every possible proof for all manner of philosophical systems and ideas or, equally, to contradict every argument. He always described himself as a sceptic. I once heard him make what is in some ways a rather terrible statement: Well, all philosophy is, in the end, no more than a very beautiful way of playing with ideas!

Having often watched the sparkling intelligence of Müllner's play with ideas, I found it most interesting to observe how he could never be pinned down on any particular point since he had never admitted anything specific. When someone else expressed disagreement with some world view or other, he would then lovingly put forward every possible argument in favour of that world view, even though, perhaps a few days earlier, he had himself ingeniously condemned it down to the ground. He was an exceedingly interesting thinker, in fact in a sense even one of the most important philosophers of our age. And why he was basically like this is also interesting. Apart from having a thorough knowledge about the philosophical progress of humanity he was also a Catholic priest, and essentially he always wanted to remain a good Catholic priest even though latterly he was a professor at the University of Vienna.

The way in which he immersed himself in the Catholic way of thinking brought it about in some measure that the religious fervour of his immersion in certain trains of thought made everything else in the world appear to him to be a mere playing with ideas. Yet it was his Catholic way of thinking which prevented him from extricating himself from his doubts. He was too great to remain within the merely dogmatic aspect of Catholicism and yet the Catholicism was too strong within him to allow him to rise to a truly spiritual way of scientifically comprehending reality. It is most interesting to observe a soul like this, a soul that has come to the point where one can study what would be needed to enable such an individual to arrive at reality. For of course this exceedingly perspicacious man was quite aware that he was not capable of grasping reality.

Even in ancient Greece it was possible to state what the point of departure would be for a healthy way of thinking which wants to reach reality. And that statement already put forward in ancient Greece is surely still valid today, namely that: All study undertaken by human beings must come about on the basis of amazement.[6] Let us, my dear friends, look at this in a positive light! Let us regard as something positive the fact that a soul striving to reach the truth must have within it the condition of being amazed when confronted with the universe. In fully comprehending the power of that Greek statement we are able to say: Regardless of the other reasons leading a person to search and ponder, when his point of departure is amazement about the realities of the world, then it will be akin to sowing a seed in the ground out of which a plant then grows. In a certain sense all knowledge must grow out of the seed of amazement.

The matter is different when someone does not have amazement as his point of departure but rather, perhaps, some sort of principles hammered into him in his youth by well-meaning teachers, principles which have made a philosopher of him; or when the circumstances of his upbringing meant that it was customary to enter into a philosophical way of thinking under the influence of prevailing attitudes. It is also well known that the final examinations in philosophy are the easiest of all. In short, there are hundreds and thousands of paths which lead to philosophy without involving amazement. All such points of departure lead to a way of living with the truth which resembles making a plant out of papier mâché instead of growing one from seed.

This is an entirely valid comparison because all true knowledge with any prospect of comprehending the riddles of the universe must grow out of the seed of amazement. However sagacious a thinker might be, even one who suffers from a kind of exuberance of sagacity will get nowhere if he has never passed through the stage of amazement. He will devise sagacious, clever concatenations of ideas none of which will be incorrect; but that which is correct does not necessarily have to lead to reality. Before we begin to think, before we even set our thinking in motion, it is essential that we pass through the state of amazement, for a kind of thinking which progresses without the state of amazement will, after all, remain a mere playing with ideas. Thinking simply must originate from amazement.

And this is not all; even this is insufficient. Although thinking must originate in amazement, there may be a person who through his karma has a turn of mind which is quite sagacious, but if he develops this sagacity alone, then any initial amazement is no help. If after some initial amazement he proceeds to develop his thinking merely through thinking, he will be unable to progress to finding reality. Of course I am not saying that a person must become thoughtless or that thinking is harmful. This is a view which is rather prevalent, even in theosophical circles where thinking is regarded as bad and damaging even by people who say that thinking must emanate from amazement. Once one has begun to think and is able to list the seven principles of the human being and so on,[7] it is not necessary to cease thinking, for thinking must continue.

But after amazement has set in another state of soul must be achieved, and that is the state of reverence for that which is approached by thinking. After the state of amazement the state of reverence, of awe, must be attained. And any thinking which emancipates itself from reverence, from an awed view of what is revealed by thinking, will be unable to penetrate through to reality. Thinking must never be permitted to trip, light-footed, around the world. Once it has moved beyond the state of amazement it must become rooted in the feeling of reverence for the grounds of the universe.

Here the path of knowledge becomes very much the antithesis of what we today speak of as science, for this is where we might say to a person standing with his test tubes in a laboratory analysing substances and synthesizing others: This is not the way to arrive at the truth! You can analyse and synthesize as much as you like, but the results are merely facts! You are approaching the facts of the world without respect, without reverence. You should stand before the reactions in your test tube with the respect and reverence of a priest before the altar.

But what would be that person's reply nowadays? He would most probably laugh in your face, be full of derision, because from their point of view modern-day scientists are quite unable to see any connection between reverence on the one hand and truth or knowledge on the other. If he did not laugh at you, he would at best concede: I am truly thrilled by what goes on in my test tubes, but you cannot convince a sensible individual that my enthusiasm is anything other than my own private affair and has nothing to do with the discovery of truth. This is the second stage.

But even after attaining some degree of reverence, if a person continued to proceed as before merely with his thinking, he would again reach something unreal and be unable to make progress. His discoveries would be correct and, because he would have taken the first two steps, that correctness would be founded on certain firm principles. But he would nevertheless soon begin to feel uncertain once more. The reason for this is that it is necessary for a third stage to be reached in our soul. Having become sufficiently immersed in amazement and reverence, the third stage might be described as feeling oneself to be in wisdom-filled harmony with the laws of the universe.

You see, feeling oneself to be in wisdom-filled harmony with the laws of the universe can only be attained once one has in some way fully understood how meaningless mere thinking is. One must tell oneself over and over again that a person who relies solely on the correctness of thinking, whether in confirming or denying something, is in the same situation as the small boy who quite correctly calculated the number of rolls. If he had been able to tell himself: What I have worked out may very well be correct, but I must not rely on my correct thinking but should instead search for the truth and enter into reality—then he would have discovered something higher than correctness, namely the village custom of adding a further roll when five are purchased. He would have discovered that one must turn away from oneself and enter fully into the world, and that correct thinking has no bearing on reality.

However, it is not at all easy to enter into wisdom-filled harmony with reality. If it were easy, dear friends, then neither you nor anyone else would ever have experienced being seduced by Lucifer. For in truth it was indeed the intention of the divine guides of the world that human beings should be endowed with the ability to distinguish between good and evil, to gain knowledge, to eat from the tree of knowledge. But this was to have come about much later. The mistake human beings made was to want to attain such knowledge too soon, to want to distinguish between good and evil too soon. It was Lucifer's seduction which made them want what should only have come about later on. This is how such inadequate knowledge has come about, knowledge for which human beings should have been obliged to strive and which is now like a premature birth by comparison with a child carried to full term.

It was the Gnostics of old—and we can sense how right they were—who said that the knowledge accompanying human beings from one incarnation to the next is a premature birth, an ektroma[8]—they used this very word—because humanity could not wait until whatever should have led to genuine knowledge had been properly experienced. In other words, periods of time should have been allowed to elapse during which certain states of soul would have ripened within the human being which would then have enabled true knowledge to arise. Humanity is still committing this original sin today, for if we were to refrain from committing it we would be in less of a hurry to regard one fact or another as the truth but would instead seek to gain in maturity in order to comprehend certain truths.

Again, people today would be puzzled to be told: You think you perfectly understand the theorem of Pythagoras. But if you really wanted to comprehend in all its mysterious significance the theorem that the square on the hypotenuse of a right-angled triangle is equal to the sum of the squares on the other two sides ... or let us take a simpler example: If you want to comprehend the fact that $3 \times 3 = 9$, you will first need to have a variety of experiences in your soul! And a person today would be even more amused to be told: You will only truly comprehend this when you have brought yourself into harmony with the laws of the universe which have ordered things in such a way as to make the laws of mathematics appear to us as they do. People today are still committing the original sin when they believe that they can comprehend everything at every stage while paying no attention to the fact that they first need to have certain experiences in order to comprehend something; they must realize that they have to feel inwardly supported by the understanding that however many firm judgements they may make they can achieve nothing in matters of reality.

This belongs to the third stage which I want to describe. However much effort we put into making a judgement, errors can always arise. A correct judgement only results if we have attained a certain degree of maturity, if we have waited until the judgement itself leaps towards us. It is not when we make the effort to reach a judgement but when we make the effort to be ready for the judgement that it comes towards us; and then the judgement has something to do with reality. However much effort you devote to forming a correct judgement, you can never be sure that this inner effort will achieve a competent judgement. You can only hope to arrive at a correct judgement if you devote every care to becoming ever more and more mature, by as it were waiting for the correct judgements to come to you through the revelations which enter into you because you have become mature. One can have the most remarkable experiences in this way. A person who is quick and ready with a judgement will, of course, think: If someone has fallen into the water and been pulled out dead, he must have drowned. But a person who has grown wise and mature through the experiences in his life will know that in every individual case a generalized judgement is meaningless. He will know that in every single instance he encounters he must allow the judgement to arise out of the facts he sees played out before his eyes. Life itself can show how true this is.

Suppose a person says something but that you have a different opinion. You can point out that what he is saying is wrong. Your judgement can be entirely different from his. Indeed, what he says and what you say might both be wrong. Both judgements might be right or both might be wrong. At this third stage it will not be relevant to you that one person forms a judgement which differs from that of another. That is not what is relevant. A wise person will always hold back with his judgement in order not to become too involved with it; he will even hold back when he is aware that he might indeed be right—he will hold back as a kind of experiment, as though trying it out. Or if someone tells you something today and then in two months' time says the opposite, there is no need for you to get involved since you have nothing whatever to do with the two facts. If you let the two facts work upon you there is no need for you to make a contradiction since the two make their own contradiction. Here it is not you but the world around you which forms the judgement. And it is only at this point that the wise person begins to judge.

It is interesting to note that if one lacks the concept about wisdom making judgements one will never know, for instance, how Goethe carried out his scientific studies. That is why Goethe made the interesting statement[9]—you will find it in my introduction to Goethe's scientific works—that one should never form judgements or hypotheses about external phenomena because the phenomena themselves are the theories, they themselves give expression to their ideas if one has made oneself mature enough to allow them to work upon one in the right way. It is not a matter of making an effort to squeeze out of one's soul what one considers to be correct; one must be prepared for the judgement to leap towards one out of the facts themselves. Our relationship with thinking must not be to make thinking the judge of things but to allow it to be an instrument through which the things speak to us. That is what is meant by being in harmony with the things.

Once we have come to grips with this third state it is still not permissible for thinking to stand on its own feet, for we are now reaching what is in a certain way the loftiest state of soul to be attained if we want to reach the truth. This is the state which is well described by the word acquiescence. Amazement, reverence, wisdom-filled harmony with the world's phenomena, acquiescence to the course of the world—these are the stages through which we have to pass, stages which must always run parallel with thinking and which thinking must never be permitted to forsake, for otherwise thinking will only achieve what is correct but not what is true. Let us now pause at the place we have reached thus far, to which we have risen via amazement, reverence and wisdom-filled harmony with the world's phenomena, arriving at what we have described as acquiescence, which we have not yet explained but about which we shall continue to speak tomorrow. Let us retain our hold on acquiescence, but let us also retain our hold on the question already raised: Why is it necessary to be merely intellectual in order to refute spiritual science? We shall proceed with these two questions tomorrow.

LECTURE 2

HANOVER, 28 DECEMBER 1911

IN our considerations yesterday we reached the state of soul which we described as acquiescence. We saw that it is as yet the highest of the soul states to be attained if thinking, what we ordinarily describe as knowledge, is to enter into reality, if thinking is to have any connection with genuine reality—thinking, in other words, that has raised itself through the states of soul firstly of amazement, then of reverence towards the world of reality, and then what we termed a wisdom-filled harmony with the world's phenomena. A thinking incapable of raising itself in addition into the soul-region characterized as acquiescence would not be capable of reaching reality. This acquiescence can only be attained by means of endeavouring energetically to become ever and again aware of the incompetence of mere thinking, and by means also of endeavouring to create a lively and energetic mood which continuously says to us: You should not expect your thinking to provide you with knowledge of what is true, to give you knowledge of the truth; you should initially only expect your thinking to educate you, to bring you up. It is exceedingly important to develop within us this mood of sensing that our thinking educates us. You see, if you really carry this principle through in a practical way you will be able to reach beyond a good deal more than you would normally expect.

I suspect that not very many of you have made a thorough study of the philosopher Kant. But this would not have been necessary anyway. All that needs to be said at present is that in Kant's most important, most pioneering work, *Critique of Pure Reason*, there is always a for and an against for every proof. For example, let us take the sentence stating that the world had its beginning in time.[10] To this he might add on the next page the statement that the world has existed forever, in all eternity. Kant puts forward valid arguments in favour of each of these statements even though they are obviously contradictory. In other words, he proves that the world had a beginning and that the world did not have a beginning. Kant describes these statements as an antinomy which he is using in order to demonstrate the limitations of the human capacity for knowledge; he wants to show that human beings must of necessity arrive at such contradictory argumentations.

The fact is that as long as we are of the opinion that we can reach the truth by means of thinking, by means of working with concepts, by means of, let's say, thinking about experiences, in other words as long as we hope to arrive at a consensus of objective realities, as long as this is our belief it will be very dreadful for us if we are shown that each of two opposites can be proven to be true. How can such proofs lead us to reality! However, if we have trained ourselves to realize that at the very point where decisiveness should be crucial thinking can have nothing to say about reality, if we have energetically trained ourselves to regard thinking merely as a means towards achieving wisdom, as a means to be taken in hand for the purpose of educating ourselves towards wisdom, then we shall not be disturbed by finding that first one thing and then its opposite can be proven.

Once we have reached this point we will soon notice that, with regard to working on concepts, reality can have no effect on us and thus we can work among the concepts and ideas in utter freedom and in this way educate ourselves. If we were to be constantly corrected by reality then working on the concepts would not be a means towards educating ourselves in freedom. Take good account of the fact that working on our concepts only presents us with an effective and free means of educating ourselves if we do not permit reality to interfere with our work.

What do we mean by saying it will not interfere with our work? How would reality interfere in our free work on the concepts? We can to some extent imagine such interference if we hypothetically confront our human thinking with divine thinking—and we shall see later that this need not remain hypothetical. We can say to ourselves: In the first instance we cannot conceive of divine thinking having nothing to do with reality; we can only conceive that divine thinking—hypothetically at first—most certainly does have something to do with reality. This indicates something most important, namely that if a human being makes a mistake in his thinking it is merely a mistake, but nothing too dreadful. And if he subsequently realizes that he has made a mistake he can correct it, thus contributing to his own self-knowledge and making himself wiser. But now consider divine thinking: If divine thinking is correct something comes about. But if divine thinking is incorrect, then something is damaged or destroyed.

So if we possessed divine thinking, whenever we formed a false concept we would set in train a destructive process, first in our astral body, then in our ether body and thence also in our physical body. The consequence of a false concept—if we had effective divine thinking, if our thinking were related in some way with reality—would be to set in train something inwardly resembling a slight withering in some part of our body, a process of ossification. Therefore we would certainly have to make as few errors as possible for otherwise we would soon have made so many mistakes that our body would become shrivelled and disintegrate completely; we would soon have worn it down completely by transposing our mistaken thinking into reality. We are in truth able to maintain ourselves within reality only because our thinking is prevented from interfering with this reality. So, as things are, we can make mistake after mistake in our thinking; and if we subsequently correct these mistakes, then we have educated ourselves and grown more wise without immediately causing havoc by our mistakes. If we fill ourselves more and more with the moral power of such a thought, the result will be that we eventually resign ourselves to no longer wanting to apply thinking at decisive points in our lives in order to gain knowledge about external matters.

This sounds strange, does it not! And initially it may seem impossible to put such a thing into practice. And yet although we cannot practise it entirely, we can at least carry it out to some extent. In the way we are as human beings we cannot, in our world, completely break the habit of forming judgements about things. Indeed we do have to form judgements—and in these lectures we shall come to see why. We have to do something for our life, for the way we live our life, which does not actually penetrate right into the depths of reality. We do have to form judgements, but through wisely educating ourselves we should ensure that in all our judging we practise caution in the matter of considering our judgements to be true. We should constantly endeavour to keep watch on ourselves and realize that wherever we apply our discernment we are in fact feeling our way in the dark so that there is always a possibility of being mistaken.

This is very difficult for those cocksure individuals who imagine that they cannot make any progress at all while being expected to doubt whether any judgement they might form about anything is in fact appropriate. You only have to watch how people conduct their lives and you will see that for many the most important thing is to say in any situation: I believe this, I believe that; or when they see something, they say: I don't approve of this, I do approve of that, and so on. If one does not wish to be one of those cocksure individuals, these are the habits one must break if one wants to approach reality in one's life of soul.

The important thing, then, is to develop an attitude of mind which might be characterized thus: Well, since I have to live my life I also have to form judgements; I will make use of judgements in matters of life's practicalities but not in matters of discovering the truth. In so far as I want to discern the truth I will always keep a careful watch on myself and apply a degree of scepticism with regard to any judgement I might form.

But how can we reach the truth about any kind of thought if we are not supposed to form judgements? In one sense the answer to this question was already hinted at yesterday: We must permit the things to speak to us; we must grow ever more passive towards things and permit them to express their secrets in their own way. Much would be avoided if people refrained from judging and instead let the things express their secrets in their own way. Goethe can teach us in a wonderful way about permitting the things to express their own secrets; whenever he wants to discover the truth about something he forbids himself to form judgements and permits the things to tell him their secrets.

Let us imagine how one person forms judgements while another permits the things themselves to express their secrets. There is an excellent example which can illustrate this. The one who makes judgements sees, let's say, a wolf and then describes it. He reckons that there are also other animals which resemble this wolf and in this way he reaches a generalization about it. He then says to himself: In actual fact only individual wolves exist. I form the general concept of the wolf in my mind, but 'the wolf as such' does not exist; only individual wolves exist in the world. Such a person will easily form the judgement that we are involved only with individual creatures and that there is no reality in the generalized concept, in the idea of 'the wolf'. A person who comes up with such ideas would be one who is quite conspicuously one of those who form judgements. Someone, however, who allows reality to speak,[11] how will he think about the invisible aspect of the wolf, that aspect which is to be found in every wolf and which also characterizes every wolf? Well, such a person would say something like this: I compare a lamb with a wolf, or a number of lambs with a wolf; I shall not make any judgements but will simply allow the facts to speak. Well, let us then suppose that a very obvious fact takes place before this person, namely that the wolf eats the lambs. That person would then say: What formerly skipped about in the form of lambs is now in the wolf and has been subsumed into the wolf.

It is very much worth noting that this way of looking at things demonstrates what wolf-nature actually is. Following the events externally might well lead us to the judgement: If we shut the wolf away from any other food so that it eats only lambs, then surely as time goes on its metabolism will bring it about that the wolf has within it only the substance of lambs. And yet it never turns into a lamb but remains forever a wolf. In reaching the correct judgement we are thus shown quite clearly that the physicality of the wolf cannot be grasped by means of an unrealistic concept. If we learn from the world of external facts it shows us that apart from the physical aspect this wolf also has something entirely real within it which transcends the physical; it shows us that something we do not see is very much a reality, for whatever there is which does not become submerged in the physical is the very factor which causes the wolf to remain a wolf even if it eats only lambs. The purely sense-perceptible aspect of the lambs has been subsumed into the wolf.

It is difficult to be entirely clear about the difference between forming a judgement and allowing oneself to be taught by reality. But when we understand this properly, so that we use judgement solely for matters of practical life on the one hand and permit the things themselves to teach us about reality on the other, then we shall gradually enter into the mood which can tell us what is meant by acquiescence. Acquiescence is the condition of soul which does not wish to explore the truth on its own initiative but instead looks forward to the truth which will emanate from things; it is the condition which can wait until the soul is mature enough to receive one revelation or another. Judgement wants to arrive at the truth at every step. Acquiescence does not work at penetrating one truth or another by force. Acquiescence of soul works to develop itself, to educate itself; it waits calmly until a level of maturity is reached where truth streams into us through the revelations given by the things, pervading us entirely. Working patiently in order to progress in wise self-education—that is the mood of acquiescence.

Let us now place the fruits of this acquiescence before our souls. What do we achieve through proceeding with our thinking from amazement, reverence and feeling oneself in wisdom-filled harmony with reality until we arrive at the soul condition of acquiescence? What we achieve is this: When we consider the plant world in all its greenery, or the stars with their golden glory, when we look at all this without forming any judgement from within ourselves but instead permit the things to reveal themselves to us—if we have reached this mood of acquiescence, then all things are transformed for us from what they were in the world of the senses into something entirely different, something for which no word exists other than one which is taken from our very life of soul.

All things reveal themselves, and especially the world of the senses characterized here by this line (a–b); (see drawing on page 27). Imagine you are standing here (c) before the world of the senses which spreads out before you like a veil. What is characterized here in this line (a–b) represents the sounds of the sense world as they impinge on our ears, the colours and shapes which impinge on our eyes, the fragrances and tastes affecting our other organs, also with hardness and softness and so on—all this is characterized by this line. This line is the world of the senses.

And it is in this world of the senses that we apply our ability to form judgements. So how do the external sciences come about? They come about because they, the sciences, make contact with the world of the senses and because they research by various methods the laws and so on that are at work in this sense-perceptible world.

Through the whole essence of our discussions thus far we have seen that, since judgement is not a guide, this is not the way forward into the world of reality. We can approach the world of reality solely by educating our thinking through amazement, through reverence and so on. For then the world of the senses is transformed; it becomes something utterly new. And to make any progress in our approach to the essence of the sense-perceptible world it is important to make contact with this new element.

Let us assume that we have made good progress in developing this feeling, this soul condition of acquiescence, and are now approaching, let's say, the fresh, clear greenness of a meadow. Since there are no other plant colours in evidence, it is its fresh green which the meadow is showing us. If we have indeed progressed to a higher level of acquiescence in our soul we shall, when observing this meadow, have a feeling somehow akin to equilibrium—but a vibrant equilibrium resembling a gently harmonious rippling gush of water. We cannot help but bring up this picture as if by magic before our soul. And this feeling of inner liveliness will occur whenever we experience in our soul a taste, a fragrance or any other sensation. No colour, no sound exists without expressing something. Everything gives expression to something, and everything says something which urges us to react with a feeling of inner liveliness—not with a judgement but with inner liveliness. In short, we have to conclude that the entire world of the senses rises into our view as something which we can only describe as will. When we meet the world of the senses everything is streaming, all-pervading will. Please do take hold of this: Whoever has achieved acquiescence to a higher degree will discover all-pervading will in the world of the senses.

That is why a person who has developed this acquiescence within himself, even only to a lesser degree, becomes irritated when he encounters some incongruously modish colour in the street, for he cannot help but be inwardly aroused by whatever he sees around him.

He is forever linked to the whole world by a will-force which he feels within everything. He draws near to reality through being linked by will to everything represented in the world of sense. And in this way the world of sense comes to resemble an ocean of will differentiated in the most multifarious of ways. What we otherwise feel to be diffuse and scattered attains a kind of density because of this. We as it were peer behind the surface of things, we hear beyond the things and we hear streaming will all around us. For those who have read Schopenhauer[12] I might mention that he sensed this all-pervading will one-sidedly, in the world of sound only, and that is why he describes music as what one might call a differentiated effect of the will. In actual fact, though, everything in the world of the senses is all-pervading will for one who has attained acquiescence.

Once a person has learnt to perceive how will holds sway everywhere in the world of the senses he can then also press on further. He can, as it were, move beyond the world of the senses and enter into the secrets which lie behind the sense world and are otherwise out of reach for him.

In order to comprehend what is to be described next, we must first ask: By what means do we know anything at all about the world of the senses? The answer is simple: By means of our senses; by means of our ears the world of sound; by means of our eyes the world of colours and shapes, and so on. We know about the sense world through our sense organs. A person confronting the sense world in an everyday manner lets it work upon him, and forms judgements. The person who has attained acquiescence first of all lets the sense world work upon him; but then he feels how the all-pervading will at work in the things flows out towards him so that he floats in a communal ocean in which the will holds sway.

When such a person feels himself confronted by this all-pervading will, his development then drives him onward, so to speak as though of its own accord, to the next stage. Having first passed through the previous stages of feeling himself in harmony with the world's wisdom, of reverence, and of amazement, he then learns, as these previous stages work into the finally attained stage of acquiescence, how it is possible to become united with the things also with his ether body, which is in the background of his physical body.

In the will holding sway the person first becomes united with the things through his sense organs, that is through his physical body. When we see, hear, smell and so on, the consequence of this is that having attained acquiescence we feel how the all-pervading will streams into us as though through our eyes and ears; we feel how we ourselves are correlated with the things. Behind the physical eye, however, there exists the ether body of the eye, and behind the physical ear there is the ether body of the ear. Our ether body permeates us entirely.

And so just as the physical body becomes united through the all-pervading will with the things of the sense world, so does our ether body also become united with them. But when the ether body becomes united with the things, we become enveloped in an entirely new way of viewing what we see. The world is then transformed in a far greater degree than is the case when we progress from the sense appearance to the all-pervading will. When we become united with the things with our ether body, these things of the world make an impression on us which renders us unable to leave them as they are, for they become changed for us when we enter into a relationship with them.

Let us consider a person who has passed through the soul state of acquiescence. He looks at a green, sap-filled leaf of a plant and then directs the attention of his soul to this leaf. He cannot leave this green, sap-filled leaf as it is, for at the very moment when he looks at it he feels that it is growing beyond itself. He feels that this green, sap-filled leaf has within it the possibility of becoming something entirely different. When you consider the green leaf you know that bit by bit it will grow upwards and become the coloured petal of a flower. The plant as a whole is actually a transformed leaf. You can learn this from Goethe's research into nature.[13]

In short, the person looking at the leaf sees that it is as yet unfinished, that it wants to progress further; he sees beyond what is evident in it. And he is so touched by the green leaf that he feels something like burgeoning life within himself. He becomes united with the green leaf and senses burgeoning life within himself. And suppose he looks at the withered bark of a tree. He cannot become united with the withered tree bark in any other way than by being overcome by a mood of death. He sees less in the withered bark than it actually represents. Someone who only contemplates the sensual illusion of the bark will marvel at it and it will please him. He is then not seeing the shrivelling aspect of the lifeless tree bark which pierces the soul and fills it with thoughts of death.

When such a uniting of the ether body with the things occurs, there is nothing in the world which does not cause either feelings of growing, of becoming and sprouting or else feelings of decay and decomposition. It is in this way that we look into the things.

Suppose, for example, that a person, having reached the stage of acquiescence in his self-development, were to turn his attention to the human larynx. The human larynx appears to such a person in an extraordinary way as an organ which is at the very beginning of what it will become because it has a great future ahead of it. One feels this immediately because the larynx itself expresses it as its own truth: it is like a seed and not a fruit or something in the process of withering away. We learn from what the larynx itself tells us that something will occur in the course of human evolution. The larynx will be entirely transformed, so that whereas now it can only bring forth the word, it will one day give birth to the human being.[14] It is the future organ of birth. Just as now the larynx brings forth the word, so will it be the seed for the organ which will in the future bring forth man, the entire human being, once he has become spiritualized. This is directly shown to us by the larynx when we permit it to tell us what it is. Other organs in the human body are revealed as having long since passed the culmination of their development; we see that they will in future not be a part of the human organism at all.

Something resembling a coming into being towards the future and a dying away towards the future appears to us through this form of contemplation. Burgeoning life and decomposition, dying away, are the two things which mesh with one another when we attain this bonding of our ether body with the world of reality. This is something which will become a very arduous test for us when we have progressed a little way. Every creature we encounter will make itself felt in the way some aspects within it will give us the feeling of burgeoning and sprouting while other aspects will generate in us the feeling of dying away. These two fundamental forces will tell us all about what we are seeing behind the veil of the sense-perceptible world. What we see in this way is termed by spiritual science the world of coming into being and dying away. So by looking into the sense-perceptible world we have a view of coming into being and dying away, and what stands behind this is all-pervading wisdom.

Behind the all-pervading will is the all-pervading wisdom! I am using the expression 'all-pervading wisdom' for the simple reason that normally the wisdom which people bring to bear on their concepts is not an all-pervading wisdom but a thought-out wisdom. The wisdom we acquire by looking beyond the all-pervading will is linked with the things, and where wisdom is at work in the realm of the things it is the all-pervading wisdom which gives true expression to its workings, the wisdom which is actually present. Where it removes itself from reality, that is where dying comes about, but where it flows in, that is where coming into being arises, a beginning, a sprouting, burgeoning of life. You see, the world which we are contemplating here, which we may characterize as the second world, can be defined so that we can say about it: At first we are contemplating the world of the senses A and the all-pervading wisdom B which exists behind the sense world. It is out of this that the substance of our ether body is taken. What we see out there as the all-pervading wisdom is what we perceive in our own ether body. And what we see in our own physical body is not solely what is sense-perceptible but also all-pervading will, because it is all-pervading will which we see everywhere in our world of sense.

This is what is so striking: When, having attained acquiescence, we meet and contemplate another person, then his bodily colouration, be it reddish or yellowish or greenish, does not merely appear to us as being reddish or yellowish or greenish. We become, in effect, as though united with the redness of his cheeks; we become united with the reality in which the all-pervading will is living. In other words we see everything alive and at work within him shooting across to us because of the redness of his cheeks. Those who are themselves in tune with noticing ruddy cheeks will say: A red-cheeked person is the only healthy one. You see, we approach the person himself in such a way that we are able to see the all-pervading will in him. Therefore we can say: Our physical body, diagrammatically indicated here by this circle, is taken from the world A, from the world of the all-pervading will—the physical body! In contrast, our ether body, which I suggest here by this second circle, is taken from the world of all-pervading wisdom, the world indicated by the letter B. This, then, is a characterization of the connection of the world of all-pervading wisdom, as it spreads out all around, with our own ether body—and the connection of the world of all-pervading will, as it spreads out all around, with our own physical body.

In everyday life we are deprived of the ability to know about a connection between the one and the other. As you can see, in the way I have made this drawing it shows that there is a direct connection between the external world of the senses and our physical body, and between the world of all-pervading wisdom and our ether body. Associations exist here. But this connection is hidden from us; we can have no influence on it. Why do we have no influence? Well, this is because there could be an occasion when our thoughts, and our whole life in the way we develop it in our soul as our life of judgement, could be, let's say, not unharmful for our own everyday reality.

For everyday life, when we are awake, certain good gods have ensured

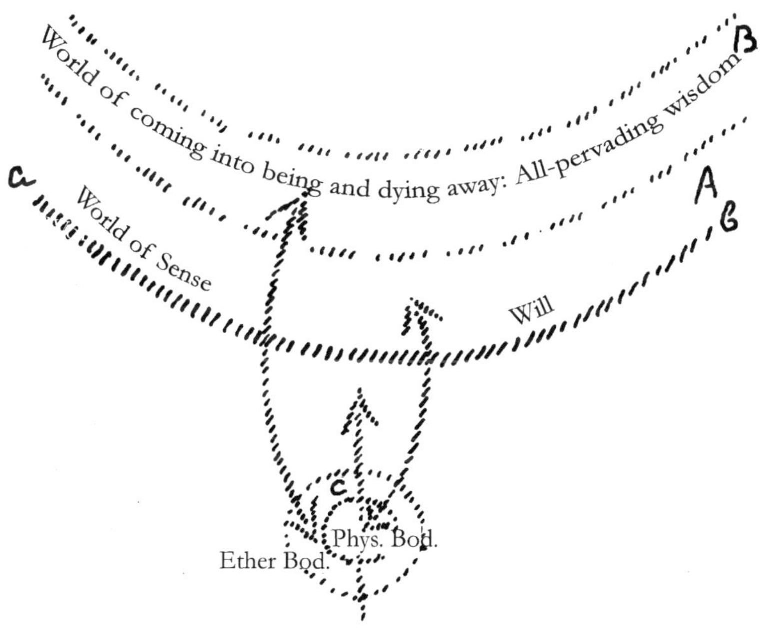

that our thoughts do not have too disastrous an effect on our own reality; they have deprived us of the power our thoughts could have over our physical body and over our ether body, for if they had not done so the world would be in a very sorry state. Let me emphasize this again: If thoughts were really to have the significance in the human world which they do have in truth as divine thoughts, then with every error he made a person would set in train a small process of withering within himself, and soon he would dry up entirely. And as for telling a lie! If a person were to burn up the corresponding portion of his brain with every lie, which is what would happen if he were to have any influence in the world as far as truth is concerned, he would soon see how long his brain could hold out.

Those good gods have, so to speak, withdrawn from our souls any power over our ether body and our physical body. But this cannot be the case all the time. If it were permanently not possible for our soul to exercise any influence over our physical and ether body, then we would very soon have used up all the forces in our physical and ether body and our life would be very short. As we shall see during the course of these lectures, there are forces in our soul which must flow into our physical and ether body, forces which we need in the latter. So at certain times streams of force must flow from our soul into the ether body and the physical body. This takes place during the night while we are asleep. That is when the forces we need in order to banish tiredness flow from the universe via a detour through our 'I' and our astral body. Then there is indeed this living connection of the world of will and the world of wisdom with our physical and ether body. It is into these worlds that our astral body and our 'I' disappear while we sleep. They enter there and that is where they create centres of attraction for the substances which must now flow from the world of wisdom into the ether body and from the world of the all-pervading will into the physical body.

This has to take place during the night. If we were really to be conscious during this process, you would soon see how this in-flowing would proceed! If we were to be conscious with all our errors and vices and with all the ills and so on which we commit in the world, then all this would be an extraordinary kind of trap for the forces which ought to flow in. Horrendous destructions would be visited on our ether body and our physical body through what we would send from our 'I' and our astral body into our physical and our ether body out of the world of all-pervading wisdom and the world of all-pervading will.

That is why those good gods made sure that we cannot be consciously present when the proper force has to flow into our physical and our ether body during the night. For this circumstance they have suppressed our consciousness during sleep so that we cannot cause the damage with our thoughts which we would otherwise certainly cause. This is also what gives rise to the greatest pain when we are endeavouring to reach higher worlds on the path of knowledge if we are making a great effort in this respect. In the description in *How to Know Higher Worlds*[15] you will have seen how our life during the night, our life during sleep, is used in a specific way to help us ascend from external reality to the higher realms. When we begin to illuminate our sleep consciousness with knowledge and experiences, we must indeed see how to set about properly excluding from our consciousness all sources of destruction which might affect our physical and our ether body.

This is what makes it absolutely necessary to know ourselves thoroughly when endeavouring to reach the higher realms. If we really know ourselves very thoroughly we usually stop loving ourselves. Self-love usually ceases when we begin to know ourselves. This loving of oneself, which is always present in those who have not attained self-knowledge (for it is erroneous to believe that one does not love oneself, indeed one loves oneself more than anything else in the world), this self-love must have been overcome if one is to exclude oneself, for this is what is necessary. When aiming for higher realms we have to say: If this is what I am like, I will have to eliminate myself. We have already achieved a great deal by attaining acquiescence, but we must not love ourselves at all. We must always be capable of feeling: I must push myself aside. If I am unable to push to one side all the things I otherwise love about myself, all those errors, all that is mean-minded, the prejudices, sympathies, antipathies and so on, if I do not push all this to one side, then, as I ascend, certain forces will become mingled with what ought to enter into me so that I may become clairvoyant. They flow into my physical and ether body, and there are then so many errors, so many destructive processes.

If we have no consciousness during sleep, if we are unable to ascend into the worlds of clairvoyance, then good gods prevent these forces from entering into the streams of the world of all-pervading will and the world of all-pervading wisdom and thence into our physical and ether bodies. But if we carry our consciousness up into the world of clairvoyance no gods protect us any longer—for the very protection they give us consists in taking away our consciousness. So then it is up to us to remove all those prejudices, sympathies, antipathies and so on ourselves. All this has to be pushed to one side; for if we still harbour any kind of self-love, any kind of wishes that are personal to us, if we are still capable of reaching some judgement or other for personal reasons, then all this causes damage to our health, to our physical body and our ether body while we proceed to ascend further into the higher worlds.

It is immensely important to keep a very firm watch on this. We must convince ourselves how significant it is that in ordinary daytime life we cannot exercise any influence over our physical and ether bodies—because when we are within our physical and ether bodies our thoughts have nothing whatever to do with reality and can therefore not have any decisive influence on it. During the night, however, they can indeed have a decisive influence on reality. Every false thought would destroy the physical and the ether body. We would see before us everything that has just been described.

The world of the senses would appear to us as an ocean of all-pervading will. And behind this the wisdom which builds the world would appear working through the will, whipping it hither and thither. It would show itself as the force which, with the breaking of its waves, continuously brings about the processes of coming into being and fading away, the processes of birth and death. It is the world of truth into which we look, the world of all-pervading will and the world of all-pervading wisdom; and the latter is the world of coming into being and dying away, of continuous births and continuous deaths. It is the world which is our own and which it is immensely important to recognize. For once we have recognized it we begin to see in it an important means of attaining ever higher and higher acquiescence because we find ourselves interwoven within perpetual births and perpetual deaths. In whatever we do we are in some way within the coming into being and the dying away. And something which is good becomes for us something about which we do not merely say: This is good, this fills me with sympathy. No, we now begin to know: The good is something creative in the universe, something which everywhere signifies the world of coming into being. And about the world of evil we feel everywhere that it is an outpouring of decay.

This is an important transition to a new view of the world, one in which evil can surely be felt to be the stifling angel of death striding through the world, and in which good can surely be felt to be the creator of perpetual births of worlds both great and small. To those who comprehend such a description, spiritual science shall give an inkling of how one's view of the world can become more and more profound through the direct feeling: The world of good and the world of evil are not merely what they appear to be in external *maya* where with our ability to form judgements we confront evil and good merely in finding the one to be sympathetic and the other antipathetic. No, the world of good is the world of creativity, and evil is the stifling angel advancing across the world with his scythe. And with every evil we commit we help the stifling angel, we take his scythe into our own hands and participate in the processes of death and decay. The concepts we glean from spiritual foundations give strength to our whole view of the world. This is what is strong, and it is what human beings must from now on take up in the future development of civilization and culture, for this is what they will need. Until now good gods have taken care of us, but in our fifth post-Atlantean period the time has come when our destinies, when good and evil are once more in our own hands. And that is why it is necessary for human beings to know the meaning of good in its creativity and of evil as a death-dealing principle.

Lecture 3

HANOVER, 29 DECEMBER 1911

In yesterday's lecture we saw how our physical body is connected with our sense-perceptible world. We were shown that the human physical body consists, so to speak, of the matter we also find in the external, sense-perceptible world, and which was also described yesterday as will. We can say, therefore, that in the outer sense-perceptible world there is all-pervading will, and that in truth there is also all-pervading will in the human physical body. And in this respect the human body is a part of the external world of the senses. We found that behind the sense-perceptible world there lies the world of coming into being and dying away, and we also found that in its true nature this can be described as all-pervading wisdom. And in addition we found that our human ether body, too, is made from the substance of the all-pervading wisdom. Within the human ether body and physical body there is also what we call the astral body and the 'I'. The human being as a whole here on the earth consists of physical body, ether body, astral body and 'I'.

We have now reached the moment in our considerations when it will be necessary to introduce a subject which may be somewhat difficult to comprehend, but it will lead us very profoundly into an understanding of the world and especially of the human being. We can assume as our starting point that physical body, ether body, astral body and 'I' have to be combined in some way. However, someone who, through clairvoyance, can examine this combination of the four members of the human being will have a particular impression—and we shall see how important it is to examine this impression—namely that the combination of these four elements of human nature is irregular. At some point disorder must have entered into this combination. When examining the four members of the human being one gains the impression that they are not arranged one within another as they should be but are instead mingled in a disorderly way. At some point disorder occurred. This is the impression one gains. When touching on the mysteries of life we can realize what infinite depths are contained in occult, religious archives when they are correctly interpreted.

As we proceed we shall see what is meant by this disorder, this irregularity which is marvellously expressed in the Bible with the words Lucifer speaks to the human being when he wants to lead him astray: Your eyes shall be opened and ye shall . . . know good and evil.[16] These words are immensely profound. They do not simply mean that the eyes will be opened, for the eyes here represent all the senses together. If we understand Lucifer's words correctly we can translate them as follows: All your senses will work in ways which would not be intended if you wanted to follow only the gods and not me also—meaning Lucifer. The senses work in a different manner on account of Lucifer's intervention. It is exceedingly difficult for people today to imagine how the senses work, and I shall have to make a good many grotesque explanations in order to show you how the senses would really work if disorder had not entered into the combination of the four elements of the human being through Lucifer. Grotesque explanations are needed because people as they are today cannot imagine that something other than what they actually experience would have been correct from the beginning.

What could be more natural or obvious today for someone asking what our eyes are for than to receive the reply: Obviously, they are for seeing. And you could say it would be his right to regard a person who says they are not for seeing as a fool! Yet from the very beginning of earth's evolution human eyes were not intended for seeing. They only became organs for seeing as a consequence of Lucifer's seduction. The actual faculty of sight for the human being was not intended to pass out through the eye towards the so-called things; it was intended to reach only as far as the eye so that with every activity of seeing—if things had proceeded in accordance with the original intentions of the gods—human beings were supposed to become directly aware of their eyes;

instead of seeing something external they were supposed to experience their eyes. They were supposed to become aware of the activity as such at work within their eyes, whereas nowadays they are not aware of the activity of seeing except in its result, namely an encounter with some kind of external object. Human beings were supposed to become entangled in the activity much sooner than the moment when their seeing met an object. They were supposed to become aware of it in the eyes themselves through feeling their activity.[17]

Nowadays this is almost impossible in the case of the eyes unless a person has undergone a specific spiritual development. People can do it with their hands since they can at least distinguish whether they are grasping an object or merely waving their hand about to no purpose; so in the case of the hands a person can become aware of the hands' activity. But if people's power of sight is guided only by their eyes, they see nothing. This is how things are now, but originally it was not the intention. Originally, with the eyes—or indeed the ears or any other sense organ—a person was to have experienced the all-pervading will; he was to have been immersed in the all-pervading will, realizing that this was so in the specific way it affected his eyes. It was to have been similar in the case of the eyes as it is with the hands. When you take hold of something you feel that it is hard if you find it difficult to get the better of it, and that it is soft if you can easily crush it. You feel what you are doing with your hand. This would be the case with the eyes as well; you would only feel the eyes, only directly experience the eyes as being directly linked with the all-pervading will, if your ether body were correctly inserted into your physical body.

But now our ether body is not correctly inserted into our physical body. This is the peculiarity, that the ether body is not correctly inserted into the physical body. And this is only one example of the disorder within the human being. Not one of the human being's elements is correctly inserted into the others; everything in the human being is in disarray. If there had been no luciferic influence at work at the starting point of earthly evolution, all the insertions of the four members of the human being would have been different. This is what we must begin to understand; that something quite specific was brought about by the disorder which occurred through the influence of Lucifer on the bringing together of the four members of human nature.

Let us explain this as follows, after first making a chart as an aid (see p. 44). We can begin with the relationship of the physical body and the ether body as it is inserted within the physical body. If, as originally intended by the guiding gods, the ether body were to be poured into the physical body, the human being would hear all around him—it is difficult to find words for these things since they are not actually thus—something akin to a continuous murmuring of all-pervading will. He would hear everywhere a differentiated all-pervading will, and he would perceive some difference in the workings of the will depending on whether he was aware of focusing his eyes or his ears and so on upon the world. These organs would enable him to experience the different aspects of the will, but he would everywhere sense its murmuring. This would happen if, as we have said, the ether body were inserted into the physical body in an orderly manner as intended by the guiding gods.

However, this is not the case. The ether body is not completely within the human physical body, and so a small portion of the physical body has been left to itself. The ether body does not fully permeate the physical body, so that in a certain way the physical body possesses a preponderance of its own activity which it should not have. Thus there are parts of the human physical body which are not as completely permeated by the ether body as they should be according to the original intentions of the divine-spiritual beings who guide earthly evolution. The portions where the physical body is not permeated by the ether body in an orderly manner are those where the sense organs are formed. And it is because of this that the sense organs are shaped in the way they are today. Therefore in every sense organ there exists the highly remarkable situation in which purely physical manifestations occur which are as though excluded from the general workings of life.

Consider that you have in your eyes something which can be compared with a darkroom, a photographic apparatus, which functions in accordance with physics. It is as though a piece of the physical body had been detached from the general permeation by the ether body. And this is in fact the case. It is the same with that characteristic of the inner ear where in the inner passage there is something like a keyboard. The ether body is as though pushed back so that the physical body produces physical effects of its own which are not appropriately permeated by the ether body; hence there arise what we term the sense impressions. Colours are experienced because the ether body does not permeate the eyes in the proper manner, so that purely physical effects occur.

The same goes for all the sense organs: a preponderance of the physical body over the ether body comes about. So we can say, firstly: It is characteristic that in the relationship between the physical body and the ether body there is a preponderance of the physical body over the ether body. If this preponderance of the physical body did not exist, the whole world of the sense-perceptible as we know it today would be absent; instead we would find ourselves bound up with the surrounding world through experiencing everything as rippling, undulating all-pervading will. If this preponderance of the physical body over the ether body were not the case, however, then we would feel ourselves to be active and not passive, just as we feel ourselves to be active when we stretch out a hand. This, then, is an exceedingly interesting fact which is revealed by a higher, a spiritual observation of the human being, namely that the entire sense-perceptible world rests on the ether body being as though pushed back from the sense organs so that something is embedded in us which is purely physical world.

This brings us, secondly, to the relationship between ether body and astral body. Again it is not the case that the astral body permeates the ether body in the right way. Here there is a preponderance of the ether body over the astral body in human nature. Even with a low degree of clairvoyance one can investigate the preponderance of the ether body over the astral body. No great powers are needed for this. The fact is that without this preponderance, human beings would never be able to weep, among much else. They would be unable to weep. When one observes a weeping human being, someone secreting this peculiar saline liquid from his ocular glands, one realizes that this is a situation in which the activity of the ether body is too strong over against the inserted activity of the astral body. The human being cannot fully bring over into his ether body what he experiences astrally; the ether body has a preponderance over the astral body, and this preponderance comes to expression in the way in which the ether body works back into the physical body, squeezing tears out of it.

This is the case with all glandular secretions, with every process of glandular secretion within the human being. They are all due to a preponderance of the ether body over the astral body. And this preponderance, this disturbance of equilibrium is expressed in the way it further affects the physical body; all glandular secretions are the consequence. If this were not the case, glandular activity would not result in secretions; if the astral body were fully integrated within the ether body, the activity of the astral body would be fully expended in the inner mobility, the inner activity of the glands. The glands would squeeze nothing out of themselves but would expend themselves within themselves. No secretion of physical matter would result. So you see how mightily the consequences of the luciferic seduction express themselves to occult observation. If Lucifer had not interfered in the ordering of the world, human beings would never sweat—pardon the expression—for any activity or movement would expend itself within the relevant organ; nothing would make its way from the gland to the outside. This, then, is secondly a preponderance of the ether body over the astral body.

In order to link the specific nature of our world of sense with the first instance of preponderance, we can say: The preponderance of the physical body over the ether body is the cause of how our world of sense specifically appears to us. We can then continue by saying: The preponderance of the ether body over the astral body tells us how we feel about ourselves. The overall state of our feelings about ourselves, in so far as they are expressed in the body, arises from the preponderance of the ether body over the astral body. This preponderance brings about our subjective feelings regarding our purely bodily state, the overall feeling of our body.

But now, to continue with our considerations, we shall have to apply a different pattern. It would be easy to proceed according to the same pattern because we would simply say: Having constructed the preponderance of the physical body over the ether body followed by the preponderance of the ether body over the astral body, the third matter to consider would be the preponderance of the astral body over the 'I'.

But to do this would merely amount to setting up a chart based on purely intellectual principles, and it would lead nowhere. So we cannot continue along these lines. It is a fact that if, having learned about certain spiritual facts, one were to proceed diagrammatically in accordance with the intellect, it would lead us to something quite different from reality. One cannot continue along intellectual lines; or if one did one might proceed for a little while but then arrive at something different. So now our third consideration presupposes a reversal of preponderance, the preponderance of the astral body over the ether body. Our third consideration must again involve the relationship between the astral body and the ether body, but this time our clairvoyant observation reveals a preponderance of the astral body over the ether body.

This preponderance is indeed the most important of the observations we have undertaken thus far. You see, if I were to give you the most rough-and-ready portrayal of the human being, an entirely materialistic description, I could simply represent him, in the manner found in a good many materialistic books, as a capacious mechanism for digestion, a mechanism which eats and digests and builds its body from the substances it has taken in through eating and then distributed in a variety of ways, and so on. You will indeed find that the materialistic world view describes the human being as little more than a capacious mechanism for digesting and eating, a mechanism which takes in substances from outside and processes them inwardly, distributing them in various ways to the muscles, the bones, the sinews and so on.

A rough-and-ready view of the human being which disregards what it means to perceive a sense-perceptible world or to have an overall sensation of the body through being aware of specific glandular secretions, a view which takes account solely of how food is taken in and how its substances are transformed into blood, into the circulation of the blood and so on, such a rough-and-ready view is aware solely of the material process, and this is in fact what we mean by the physical expression of the preponderance of the astral body over the ether body. As you know, when we view the world spiritually we have to be aware of something spiritual which exists in the background of everything sense-perceptible. What is sense-perceptible is only the external semblance. So behind all the taking in and processing of food we have to see the preponderance of the astral body over the ether body. Thus the preponderance of the astral body over the ether body finds expression in the normal processes of organic life in so far as these are physical, in other words in the normal physical and organic life processes.

So we have discovered something remarkable, and I hope you will take note of it in the right way. You have to realize that what materialism often regards as the total human being and indeed what most people are chiefly concerned with—taking in food and distributing the substances to the various organs of the body—all this has been brought about by nothing other than the luciferic influence causing a displacement which resulted in a preponderance of the astral body over the ether body. What I mean is that if Lucifer had not existed at the outset of human evolution and if he had not displaced the astral and the ether body in the manner described, then human beings would not eat and digest substances in the way they do. What the materialistic view regards as the main characteristic of the human being is a purely luciferic deed; it is nothing other than the product of a displacement between astral body and ether body which has caused the astral body to gain some activity through Lucifer which gives it a preponderance over the ether body. This has been given to human beings by Lucifer, and it has brought about the human being's ability to take in physical foods. This was not originally intended for the human being; he should have had a way of existing and living at a stage where there would have been no need for him to take in physical foods.

This is awe-inspiringly expressed in the fact that Lucifer brought about what we call the expulsion from paradise. To be in paradise signifies nothing other than to be a spiritual being who has no need to take in and process physical foods. What most materialistically inclined human beings consider to be the highest delight is in fact an expulsion from paradise. Human beings have been punished not only by having to take in and process physical foods; they have been doubly punished in that most of them derive the greatest enjoyment from what in the Bible is described as the greatest loss, namely to have been driven out of paradise and therefore to be obliged to take in physical food. Human beings have changed to such an extent that for them existing outside paradise has become their greatest delight. It is remarkable that we are having to realize this, but we must.

At last we have arrived at our fourth consideration and this concerns the relationship of the 'I' with the astral body. Here the luciferic displacement brings about a preponderance of the 'I' over the activity of the astral body. What we do not have, you see, is a preponderance of the astral body over the 'I'. Instead of proceeding along the lines of a chart we must proceed according to observation, which shows us that whereas there is a double relationship between astral body and ether body we have now come to a preponderance of the 'I' over the astral body. Here the relationship of the 'I' to the astral body is not as was originally intended prior to the interference by Lucifer. The 'I' is more egoistic, it is more 'I'-ish than it should have been. It has become more egoistic, more 'I'-ish than should have been the case. This has come about through the influence of Lucifer. What happened to bring about this preponderance in the fourth of our considerations? To understand it we must take into account what the proper relationship between the 'I' and the astral body ought to be.

We can only recognize this proper relationship by, as it were, reconstructing it. As we human beings exist in the world today, living as we do under the influence of Lucifer, the relationship between the 'I' and the astral body is not correct and so there is a preponderance of the 'I'. The human being is more 'I'-ish than he ought to be—if you will excuse this coined expression which is, though, very appropriate. Actually we have already completed the consideration which shows us what the 'I' should really be like.

If we wisely and energetically and patiently train ourselves to attain what we earlier described as amazement, as the feeling of reverence for what is being explored, as the feeling of wisdom-filled harmony with the world's phenomena, and as acquiescence, then the 'I' attains the correct orderly relationship. Standing in relationship to the astral body in this way it will give the impression to an unbiased observer: Now the 'I' is correct, now it has reversed the influence that arose through Lucifer's interference. We can only restore the original relationship by training ourselves to attain the highest stage of those four qualities of soul already described.

And what does the relationship of the 'I' to the astral body then become? Well, that is the remarkable thing. You can glean what is meant by paying close attention to certain chapters in my book *How to Know Higher Worlds.*[18] In our present-day situation we are permanently bound up with our thinking, feeling and will. It is very difficult to reach a condition in our external consciousness in which we exist solely within our 'I' without being bound up with thinking, feeling and will. Try and force yourselves to comprehend the pure concept of the 'I'. The effort of grasping the pure thought of the 'I' makes our anthroposophical friends gasp when Dr Unger again and again exhorts them to think this pure thought of the 'I' without involving any of their thinking, feeling or will.[19]

This shows you how difficult it is to reach the 'I' as pure thought, quite apart from extricating it from all that thinking, feeling and will. When we are so tied up in our soul, all manner of thinking, feeling and will expressions flash through it, and desires as well. One is never separated from thinking, feeling and will with one's 'I'. But through the four conditions already described one can step outside the thinking, feeling and will and look at the 'I' as something outside oneself. We must be as indifferent to our own thoughts as we are to objects around us, so that we can no longer say: I am thinking. Instead our own thinking is like a process running its course without having anything to do with us. And the same must be the case with feeling and will.

Even thinking only a little about one's soul characteristics encourages us to say: This is something which one can imagine as an ideal, but an ideal which can be fulfilled. But we are in fact so mingled with our thinking, feeling and will that it is exceedingly difficult to extricate ourselves. It is very difficult to make our way through the world with the attitude: Here I am, walking along in the world, but I always carry with me a companion who is a part of me, one who is a kind of double of myself. The thinking, the feeling and the will carry on side by side with me. I am separate from this, I am what I am in my 'I', and I walk along side by side with this threefold companion, like three sacks which I carry with me, one of which is stuffed with my thinking, another with my feeling and the third with my will. Until we begin to practise this 'three-sack theory' we really cannot come to an adequate conception of the opposition of the 'I' to the thinking, the feeling and the will as it was originally intended to be by the divine beings before Lucifer made his approach to the human being. The human being was to have become an observer of himself, not one who experiences himself within himself.

What form did the temptation, that original temptation, take? Let us put it as simply as possible: It consisted—if I may now somewhat simplify this description—in Lucifer approaching that human 'I' which the human being was to have received in all its integrity alongside the astral body, which had already been given to him on Old Moon, and saying: See here, O man, how dull it will be to go about with this single centre of your 'I am' while being able only to look on at everything else. Surely it is far more amusing to submerge yourself in your astral body. Let me give you the power to submerge yourself in your astral body so that there is no need for you to remain one-sidedly with your 'I' while only looking on at your double; instead you may submerge yourself in it. And so that you need not feel as though you are drowning when you submerge yourself in your astral body I shall protect you by giving you some of my power.

Thus the 'I' submerged itself, and so that it should not drown it became inoculated with luciferic power. And the luciferic power thus absorbed by the human being became the preponderance of the 'I' over the astral body, an augmented 'I'-ishness which is actually a kind of luciferity.

What is this in reality? How do we encounter it in life? Initially this luciferity, this excessively large 'I'-ishness, is something we encounter through being mixed up with our thoughts, and then also with our feelings and our impulses of will. Initially it is a matter of our thoughts. If Lucifer had not approached the human being we would never have conceived the crackpot idea—please excuse the expression which is crazy for others but meaningful for us—that we possess reason, that we cherish thoughts within ourselves. Instead we would have known that the thoughts are outside us, that we must observe our thinking. The human being would have practised observation until the thought emerged, until the meaning of his thinking became clear.

This is depicted, for example, in my book *The Philosophy of Freedom.*[20] It would never have occurred to the human being to say: I must bring together all kinds of thoughts; I must form a judgement within myself. Forming judgements within ourselves, independently of what is revealed to us, is a luciferic element within us. In this way all our reasoning, in so far as we regard it as one of our characteristics, is an error. It was Lucifer's temptation which gave us the idea that we are supposed to possess reason. So now you will understand how in a certain sense this reasoning came about as a consequence of a displacement, and that our reasoning can therefore by no means be regarded as the measure for all our understanding concerning reality.

I pointed out at Karlsruhe[21] that it is entirely understandable for a person who relies on his reasoning to say: If I want to comprehend the resurrection at the Mystery of Golgotha there is nothing for it but to disregard my reasoning, for whatever my reasoning can assert must contradict the resurrection. Thus speaks the human being of the nineteenth century, and thus speaks even the liberal theologian of the nineteenth century. How can such a person expect to comprehend the Mystery of Golgotha—which is a deed lacking any connection with Lucifer, a deed which lies entirely beyond the sphere of Lucifer, a deed which came about in order to overcome the sphere of Lucifer—how can such a person ever expect to comprehend such a thing by means of his reasoning which was given to him by Lucifer!

It goes without saying that one's own reasoning can never comprehend these things. Our reasoning is a luciferic gift, so it is not suitable for comprehending things which have nothing to do with Lucifer's workings. This is the deeper meaning in this matter. If the Mystery of Golgotha were to be comprehensible to human reasoning, my dear friends, then there would have been no need for it to take place, it would have been entirely unnecessary. The very purpose for that event is to balance out the displacement which was created by luciferic influence; its intention is to cure human beings of the singular arrogance, the singular effrontery of reasoning, which expresses itself in the presumption that by employing this reason human beings can comprehend everything. This is the point at which we must grasp that reasoning as such has its limits. I have many times declared that human knowledge has its limits; however, it is reasoning as such which has its limits.

Physical body—Ether body

1. Preponderance of physical body over ether body:
World of the senses

Ether body—Astral body

2. Preponderance of ether body over astral body:
Overall bodily state of well-being

*

Astral body—Ether body

3. Preponderance of astral body over ether body:
Normal physical-organic life processes

'I'—Astral body

4. Preponderance of the 'I' over the astral body:
The 'I' interwoven with thinking, feeling and will

* This is where Lucifer and Ahriman meet

If you now look at the chart we have been developing you will say: It shows where the original disorder originated; so what must the first disorder have been in connection with the luciferic temptation? Obviously the one which we have described as the preponderance of the 'I' over the astral body.

All the influence arising from Lucifer stems from the way it gave the 'I' its luciferic power, making it mingle impurely with thinking, feeling and will, thus gaining preponderance over the astral body. From this then also arose the preponderance of the astral body over the ether body. Thus was the balance in the human being upset. It is as though the luciferic influence administered a blow to the astral body and that in its turn the astral body then passed this on and thus gained its preponderance over the ether body. But from this point on the effect does not continue. The ether body does not simply replicate the blow again. It is like hitting a buoyant ball: the blow penetrates to a certain extent but then bounces back.

We can first speak of an excess of the astral body over the ether body; but then the matter is reversed so that the ether body gains a preponderance over the astral body; it bounces back, it springs back. Here, at the number 2, the preponderance is reversed. And thence arises the preponderance of the physical body over the ether body.

These two administer a blow in reverse. Why do they do this? This happens because whereas Lucifer has been at work administering blows, here Ahriman hits back in the physical body and the ether body. So that here in the middle, where on the one hand the preponderance of the ether body over the astral body and of the physical body over the ether body is at work, while on the other hand we have the preponderance of the astral body over the ether body and of the 'I' over the astral body, Ahriman and Lucifer come up against one another. They meet here. There is a central point in man where in his own being Lucifer and Ahriman encounter one another. Here the human being has the opportunity either to swing over to the side of Lucifer and push the astral body into the ether body more deeply than is good for him or he has the opportunity to accept the impact of Ahriman and allow the ether body to be pushed more deeply into the astral body than is right and normal. These are the forces with which we have to grapple.

It will be our next task to deal with the way in which we are nowadays everywhere confronted with how certain forces work. Apart from the one instance when we spoke about the preponderance of the astral body over the ether body—where we looked at how substances are processed, how foods are taken in and processed—we have not yet come across the question of how physical substance works. What we shall have to do is investigate spiritually from a certain angle what substance, what matter actually is. This is the question with which we shall begin tomorrow.

LECTURE 4

HANOVER, 30 DECEMBER 1911

IT is relatively difficult for us to gain an idea of what we normally call 'matter'. In order to clarify spiritually the nature of matter, of substance, the main question to ask is: What is the most striking characteristic of the stuff we ordinarily call matter? Well, if we proceed without prejudice we shall find its most striking characteristic to be that it fills up space, it spreads out into space. If we have an experience in our soul, for example a feeling, or a thought, or even an impulse of will, it would never occur to us to regard these as taking up space. We can all surely see what nonsense it would be to say that one thought or another—for instance the idea of a hero—is five square metres larger than the idea of an ordinary human being. If we think this through we will soon notice that the concept of filling up space or spreading out in space cannot be applied to a state of our soul or the processes of our soul.

Another characteristic of matter, though, would be to say that it is supposed to have weight. However, this attribute of weight is not so simple, as we shall see as these lectures proceed. If we approach the world solely by looking at it, no amount of looking or contemplating will show us anything to do with weight; all we are aware of is the filling out of space, the spreading out into space.

We also know that this spreading out is usually measured by the three dimensions which we apply to space, the dimensions of height, width and depth. It is a general, an ordinary truth to say that things extend in space in accordance with the three dimensions. So we would have to recognize that this spreading out in space is the most striking characteristic of matter. When we now consider what has just been said, namely that we cannot speak about filling up space with regard to what we have in our soul, we shall have to agree that there is more to it than merely the way in which matter, substance, fills up space since there is this further observation which can also legitimately be made on the physical plane, namely that there are other processes or conditions which do not spread out in space, namely the processes or conditions of soul.

If we look at experiences of soul in the same unprejudiced way as we first looked at experiences of substance we will soon discover another characteristic of these soul experiences without which they cannot come about. And that is that they proceed in time. Even though we cannot say that a feeling or an impulse of will is five metres in length or five square metres in size, we have to agree that what we feel and think—in so far as these are experiences of soul—does run its course in time, and that there is no specific time required for these experiences, since one is earlier, another later. In short, what we experience in our soul is subject to time.

The situation is that in the reality of everything around us and everything we ourselves are, space and time relationships are mingled together. In the external world in particular, things are spread out in space while also happening one after the other in time; they require a certain amount of time. Before we begin our examination of the spiritual truths we have to ask: What is the relationship of space with time? Here in an anthroposophical cycle of lectures we are touching quite innocently upon a question which has always been one of the great questions of philosophy and about which countless thinkers have racked their brains: the relationship of time with space. With regard to this relationship between time and space which, as I just said, we are approaching quite innocently, it may not be easy for you to follow the thoughts in question since many of you are not trained philosophers. But if you make the effort to pursue such ideas you will see how infinitely fruitful they are and how, especially if you work on them in your meditation, you will be able to take them further.

It is a good idea to begin with the time which you experience in your own soul. Ask yourselves how you experience time in your own inner being; or let me be more precise by suggesting that you do not look at the time which you can tell by looking at a clock; that of course amounts merely to comparing your inner life with external events. Refrain entirely from seeing what the time is by looking at a clock or other external happenings.

Consider only how you might ask your soul: In what way is the relationship of time expressed in my own soul? Whatever the depth of your thinking and however thorough your consideration of the question might be, you will discover only one thing which is relevant to time, and this is that you are now able to grasp a thought which you have permitted to arise in you on the basis of an external observation. You look at something or you listen to something and then a thought or a conception arises in your soul. And when you question more precisely the relationship you yourself have with this conception or this thought, you have to say: While I have this thought I am myself the thought. When you try to think very deeply about this you will have to say to yourself: When I lay claim to this thought I myself am this thought in my inmost being. But while having the idea it would be a presupposition to talk in addition about 'I am' or something similar. There is no 'I am' involved in the affair while you are involved in the thought. You yourself are the thought. You would have to practise quite hard if in addition to the thought which you are having you also wanted to be something.

In the first instance you become immersed in the thoughts or feelings directly within you. Imagine a thought of this kind is aroused in you by this stick of chalk; if you take no notice of anything apart from the inner picture of the chalk arising out of your perception of it, then your own inner being is at one with this idea of the chalk. But if, having arrived at this idea, you then remember that you also saw a stick of chalk yesterday, then you are drawing a comparison between the immediate idea of the chalk and yesterday's experience of chalk. And if you have the precise thought of being immediately identified with today's chalk you will become aware that you can no longer be identified with yesterday's chalk. Yesterday's stick of chalk will have to remain as a remembered idea. So if you have truly become one with the present idea of the chalk, then the chalk of yesterday will have become something external to your inner being; so today's chalk is now your true inner being. Your memory is something to which you can look back, but juxtaposed with today's idea it is something external.

This is how it is with everything you have experienced in your soul, with the exception of the present moment. The present moment is your current inner being. You are no longer encumbered with your former experiences; they are now external to your inner being. You can make a picture of this by imagining that the present moment is the snake while everything you have already got rid of is the discarded skin of the snake. It is as though the snake discards one skin, and then another and then a third, leaving them all behind. In the same way, by comparison with your present inner being, everything else has been discarded. Thus by remembering anything you are immediately transforming something inward into something external; the idea you have of the chalk becomes something external as soon as you move on to another idea. So you are constantly working at throwing things out and making them external. You turn your back on your inner being by immediately discarding it like a skin and making it external.

This is what goes into making up the life of the soul. That which is inward continuously becomes something outward. Thus in our own inner being, in this inner spiritual process, we are able to distinguish between what is actually internal and that external something which is within the internal. We remain within, but in this inwardness we distinguish between two parts: the part which is our own inner being and that part of our inner being which has become external.

You now see that this process we have observed running its course, this process in which something inward is transformed into something outward, is what brings into being the content of our life of soul. If you think about this you will discover that what you can call your soul is everything you have experienced since that point in your early childhood when you began to remember. A person who forgets everything he has experienced would, in a way, have lost his 'I'. The ability to put our memories behind us and yet retain them like continuously discarded skins is what constitutes the reality of our soul life.

You can think of this reality of soul life as being shaped in many different ways. Please take note of the fact that moment by moment the life of soul assumes a different shape. Think of going for a walk on a beautiful starlit night, or of listening to a Beethoven symphony. In each such moment you identify within yourself a wide spectrum of your life of soul. If you leave that starlit night and enter a pitch-dark, miserable room it is like a shrivelling of your soul life. Or if the symphony falls silent then your experience of listening also shrivels. And as for going to sleep: then your life of soul shrinks to nothing until it inflates once more when you wake up again. Thus is your life of soul being continuously reshaped.

We can make a drawing of this, but it is only a symbol because we have to draw it in space whereas we are trying to depict something in time. In making a drawing we can depict multitudinous shapes. Here (a) there is a shrivelling up; and here (b) there is a spreading out. We can think of it as being shaped in manifold ways whereby here (c) we always have the content of the life of soul. This symbolic depiction—and it is merely an attempt to make visible something which is invisible—shows the inflating and deflating of the life of soul. Listening to a symphony yields a richer soul life than merely hearing one drum beating. The life of the soul, then, can be described as involving an expansion and a contraction, but not in a spatial sense. This process of expansion and contraction most certainly involves an inner spiritual movement. Movement! The life of the soul is movement.

Will Wisdom Movement Form

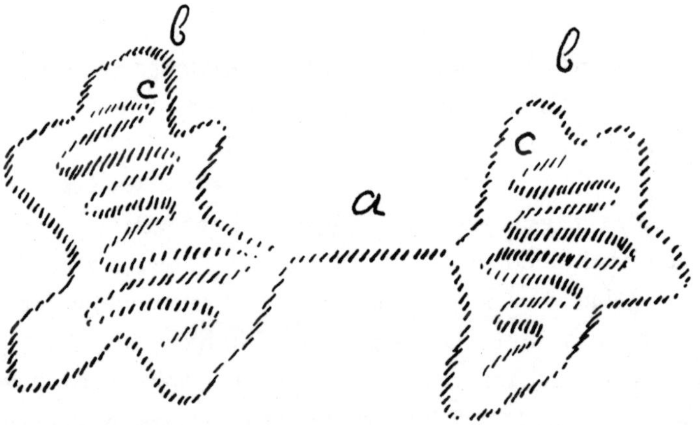

You must think of movement as such, not as something which takes place in space, but as we have described it. And this expansion and contraction yields shapes; so you have movement and an external expression of the movement in certain formations, in certain forms without, however, there being any forms in space! The forms involved are not spatial forms but forms which expand and contract, which increase and decrease the life of the soul. And what is it that lives in this expanding and contracting? Well, you could come closer to the reality of it by thinking about what must be living there. It is your feelings, your thoughts and your will impulses which live there in so far as all these are spiritual. There is a resemblance with water floating, creating forms as it moves, but spiritually of course.

And now there is only one more thing which you must imagine in order to comprehend this whole affair. We have said that thoughts live in it, ideas, feelings and impulses of will. But the will impulses are in a certain way something which is even more fundamentally necessary than the thoughts. If you consider that this soul life can be caused to move sometimes more quickly, sometimes more slowly, then you will sense inwardly that it is the will which sets these things in motion. If you stimulate your will you can cause thoughts and feelings to flow more rapidly; and if the will is sluggish, then everything runs more slowly. You need the will in order to expand the life of soul. Therefore we have the sequence: will; then everything living in feelings and ideas, which in our soul life can be understood as wisdom; then we have movement, the expansion and contraction; and finally the formation, the form which appears as the expression of movement. In the life of your soul you can distinguish quite clearly between will, wisdom, movement and form. All this lives and weaves in the life of the soul.

It is a pity that this cycle of lectures cannot be extended to last a month, for if it could we should be able to speak in more detail. Then you would see how it is possible to verify precisely what goes on in your soul, which has, you could say, will as its root and then also contains wisdom and movement and form. You will see how noteworthy it is that the sequence I have written down here for the life of soul conforms in a remarkable way with the names we have been able to allot to the succession of the hierarchies,[22] from the Spirits of Will, of Wisdom and of Movement right up to the Spirits of Form. By setting forth our own soul life like this we have, so to speak, caught hold for a fleeting moment of one aspect of the hierarchies.

The hierarchies reveal themselves in a special way within our life of soul. They show how the way in which they work is completely non-spatial. And if we had learned nothing else, we have at least discovered one important thing in what we have said, a further important characteristic of these four hierarchies—the Spirits of Will, of Wisdom, of Movement and of Form—namely that they are non-spatial. It is very important that 'form' refers to a non-spatial formation at work in soul and spirit. So when we speak of the 'forms' created by the Spirits of Form we do not mean externally spatial 'forms'; we mean these inner formations of which we only become aware inwardly and which we can grasp as our life of soul runs its course. There everything takes place solely in time. Without time you cannot comprehend any of this. Apart from giving an explanation, which is of no significance as such, you must imagine it non-spatially when you remain within the life of soul.

If the Spirits of Will were at work initially on Old Saturn, the Spirits of Wisdom on Old Sun, the Spirits of Movement on Old Moon, and the Spirits of Form on the earth, then our description of the latter—with regard to their purely inward nature—would have to say that on the earth the Spirits of Form created the human being with a form that was as yet invisible. This tallies nicely with what we discovered yesterday. At the beginning of his earthly development the Spirits of Form gave to the human being invisible, non-spatial forms. We must be aware that all the external objects we now perceive with our senses are also nothing other than an external manifestation of something spiritually inward. We must realize that behind every external, spatial, physical thing there exists something very much resembling what lives in our own soul. We do not become aware of this through our outer senses, but it exists behind what our external senses show us.

How, then, might we imagine a spiritual working which goes beyond what the Spirits of Form create non-spatially? What I mean is: If the spiritual working continues on from Will, Wisdom, Movement and Form to something beyond form, what happens then? You see, when a process in the universe has progressed until form is achieved (still entirely in the realm of spirit and soul, not in space), when this process has reached such a supersensible form, then it is only possible for the next stage to come about if the form as such breaks into fragments. And this is indeed what we see with spiritual vision. When certain forms, having been created through the influence of the Spirits of Form, reach a certain stage they are shattered. And when you look at these broken forms which arise when supersensible forms are shattered, what you are then seeing is the transition from what is supersensible to the sense-perceptible aspect of space.

That broken form is matter. When matter appears in the universe it is, for the person with spiritual vision, nothing other than smashed, shattered, exploded form. Imagine this stick of chalk to be invisible and to have this peculiar parallel-epipedic shape, and then imagine taking a hammer and smashing it to pieces so that it bursts into myriads of tiny fragments; well, then you have broken the form. And imagine that in the very moment of being smashed to bits the invisible becomes visible, then you have an image of matter coming into existence. Matter as such is spirit which develops until it attains form and then bursts, breaks, collapses in upon itself.

Matter is a heap of rubble, of spirit-rubble. It is most important to pay attention to this definition of matter being a rubble heap of spirit. Matter is, in reality, shattered spirit.

If you then continue with this train of thought you will say: Very well, but we see spatial forms such as the beautiful shapes of crystals; in crystals we are confronted with very beautiful spatial forms, and yet you are telling us that all matter is a rubble heap of spirit, that it is shattered spirit!

Well, to give you another idea, think of a stream of water trickling down (a, *see over*). Assume that it is invisible, so you cannot see it. Here (b) you place an obstacle in its way, and as it splashes down it bursts into drops (c). And imagine that the falling water is invisible but the bursting drops are visible: another image of matter coming into being. But now remove the imagined obstacle, since if it did exist it would already be matter. You must imagine that without any obstacle the matter, while spiritually gaining form, is still spiritual, for movement always precedes form. Nothing exists which has not

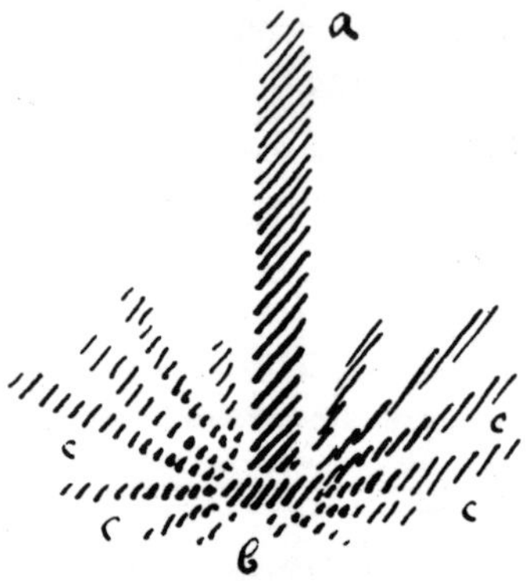

been permeated by the deeds of the Spirits of Movement. At a certain point the movement arrives at the form, loses its energy and collapses within itself.

The main idea is to imagine that something of spirit and soul beams out but only with a limited amount of momentum so that as the momentum fades it rebounds on itself and in doing so bursts. We can then say that where matter comes into existence it is based on something supersensible which has reached the limit of its effectiveness so that it then bursts. Before it bursts it still has forms spiritually within it. But after the bursting, whatever spiritual form had been there continues to work on. Where the continued working is strong, the lines of the spiritual forms continue on after the bursting. And in the lines drawn by the burst pieces as they scatter there is an expression of an after-effect. That is how crystals arise. Crystals are a subsequent creation of spiritual forms which their momentum propels backwards against the original direction.

This drawing here is almost exactly what spiritual vision gives us for hydrogen. Hydrogen looks to spiritual vision like a stream rushing in from infinity which then grows sluggish and bursts asunder. We can depict it by showing the lines overshooting and keeping their forms thus. So a particle of hydrogen looks like this, it looks like an invisible stream which arrives from the infinities of space and in the end breaks asunder like a stream scattering drops. In short, matter everywhere can be termed broken spirituality. Matter is nothing other than spirit, but spirit in a state of brokenness.

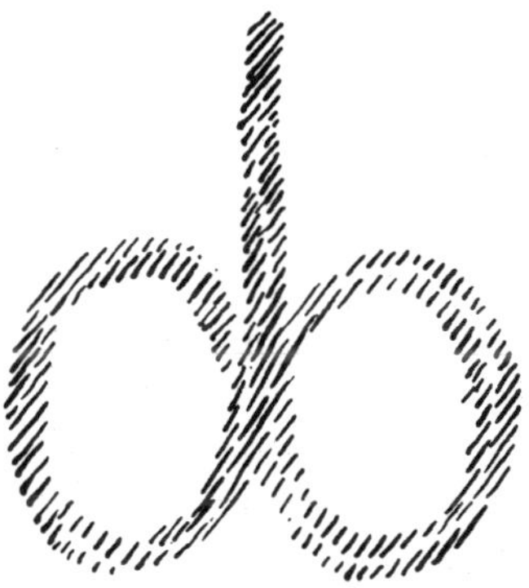

I must now present your souls with a difficult thought which is connected with what I said at the beginning. I indicated that within our inner spirit and soul we ourselves distinguish between something external and something internal. In fact, all the dimensions of space are composed of these contrasts. Thus wherever you have a dimension in space, this spatial dimension has to be seen as having a starting point somewhere; this is the internal aspect, and everything else is external. For a surface, the straight line is internal while everything else is external, and so on. Thus space is nothing other than what arises when spirit has to burst and then pass over into material existence.

Now it is exceedingly important to take note of the following. Imagine spirit bursting and shattering and thus becoming matter when there is not as yet any physical matter in existence. It bursts and shatters without meeting with any kind of previously existing external resistance. Imagine it bursting, shattering into what is, so to speak, like a vacuum. When spirit bursts into emptiness, then what comes into being is mineral matter. But now imagine spirit bursting, shattering into what is no longer a pure, virginal universe. Imagine the bursting and shattering meeting not with utter emptiness but with an existing ether substantiality. When the spirit makes its way into emptiness as it develops, then mineral matter is what arises. But suppose it develops towards an already existing ether substantiality. The bursting spirituality puffs its way into an ether body. Imagine this matter and this ether body as being already in existence. Then the bursting spirituality does not enter into the virginal nothingness of the world but into the ether body. The result is the creation not of mineral matter but of plant matter. So when spirit bursts into ether substance, the matter of vegetation is the result.

Yesterday, however, we met with a particular kind of ether substance. You remember the chart on the blackboard showing an ether body with a predominance, a preponderance over astral substance. And we said that this was the result of luciferic influences having an effect on the human being. And we found not only ether substance with a preponderance over the astral, but also a physical bodily nature with a preponderance over the ether substance of the ether body. This is what we found at first, is it not? Think now about this peculiarity which is a result solely of the luciferic influence, think about this peculiar collaboration in this imperfectly assembled human organization! Where the physical body comes upon the ether body and where the ether body is confused by the preponderance of the physical body, it is not simply the case that the spirit bursts and shatters into the ether substance; here it bursts into a body which is, indeed, an ether body, but one which is weighed down by the physical. When spirit bursts into a substance that has been prepared in this way, then the consequence is the creation of nerve substance, nerve materiality. So here we have spirit bursting into the ether bodily nature which is weighed down by physical bodily nature, and the result is nerve materiality.

We are looking at three stages of materiality: first the ordinary matter which we find here in the external world; then the matter which is found in the bodies of plants; and then the materiality of human and animal bodies as a result of irregularities. Imagine what it would take to enumerate all the various conditions regulating the many materials in the world! We saw a few irregularities yesterday brought about by the influence of Lucifer; and we saw how the ether body can have a preponderance over the astral body.

When spirit bursts into the substance of an astral body which is outweighed by the ether body, then muscle material arises. This is why both nerve material and muscle material have such an unusual appearance which cannot be compared with anything else in the external world; it is because they come into being in such a complicated way. You can see the differences when you take molten metal and splash it first into the air and then into water, and then perhaps up against something solid; this shows how complicated are the ways in which the various substantialities in the world arise.

What I mainly wanted to show you today is how deeply one must delve into existence if one truly desires to fathom these things. Let us go to where the 'I' works with a preponderance over the astral body. If spirit bursts in upon what it encounters there in this bodily irregularity which has come about through the 'I' in its 'I'-ishness outweighing the astral body, then—although in a very roundabout way—bone material comes into existence. Everything depends, as you have seen, on the way in which matter bursts asunder while being created by the spirit. Try and retain what I have been telling you even if you cannot quite follow it all with your thoughts. You will have grasped the main content, namely that matter must everywhere be seen as sparking, bursting spirit which is met by something coming towards it. Depending on what it is which comes towards it, it will spark and burst into something else, leading to the creation of various configurations of matter such as nerves, muscles, bones and so on.

A question will now be forming in your souls, and that is: What would have become of the human being if the luciferic influence had not become involved in this relationship? Yesterday we already mentioned a number of developments. But what would have taken place in this instance? Well, nerves such as we possess today would not have come into being. In their material aspect nerves only came about because of the disorder. And similarly we would have received neither bones nor muscles if the luciferic influence had not interfered. In short, we have seen various types of matter coming into being through the way in which forms pour themselves spiritually into something which is only there because of the luciferic influence. None of these muscle and nerve materials, and so on, would have arisen without the luciferic influence. We must now ask even more intensely than we did yesterday: What is the material, physical human being as a whole? As we see him externally, here on the earth, he is nothing other than the consequence of the luciferic influence. He would have neither nerves, nor muscles, nor bones in today's sense if the luciferic influence had not been present. What materialism describes is nothing other than what Lucifer has made of the human being. So in rejecting anything else, materialistic thinking is, above all, the pupilship of Lucifer.

So then, what would the human being be like if he had remained under the influence of paradise? To make it easier to build on these things in our minds tomorrow, I shall now sketch briefly what the human being would have become if the luciferic influence had not interfered. If this influence had not interfered, there would first of all, in human evolution on earth, have been what comes from the influence of the Spirits of Form. These Spirits of Form were the final spirits from among the higher hierarchies who worked in upon human beings. These Spirits of Form created form which was purely spiritual without initially any spatial aspect. What they created would have been invisible to outer eyes, for external senses cannot perceive forms which consist purely of soul elements. What would have come about is consistent with what, in *How to Know Higher Worlds*,[23] I described as imaginative knowledge. Imagination is what the Spirits of Form would initially have created. There would have been nothing sense-perceptible, but only purely supersensible Imagination.

We can look at this diagram (see Diagram 1 on page opposite) which shows approximately what would have come about; it is an image of the Imagination which the Spirits of Form created of the human being, and it would have been permeated with what previous hierarchies had also created in him. It would be permeated with what the Spirits of Movement placed in him, inner movement (Diagram 2), and it would appear to us as something which I also described in *How to Know Higher Worlds* as having been given by the knowledge arising from Inspiration, for these movements would have been recognizable purely as Inspiration. What I mean is that the whole human being would consist of Imagination, and then the next thing would come about, which is movement, Inspiration. And the Spirits of Wisdom would have given Intuition. All this would be real inner content. Here (Diagram 3) we would show Intuition, directly given by beings. And the whole would then be enveloped as though in an ovate aura appearing out of the cosmos, which would represent the Spirits of Will (Diagram 4). This would have been the supersensible nature of the human being, consisting solely of what would have been accessible to supersensible

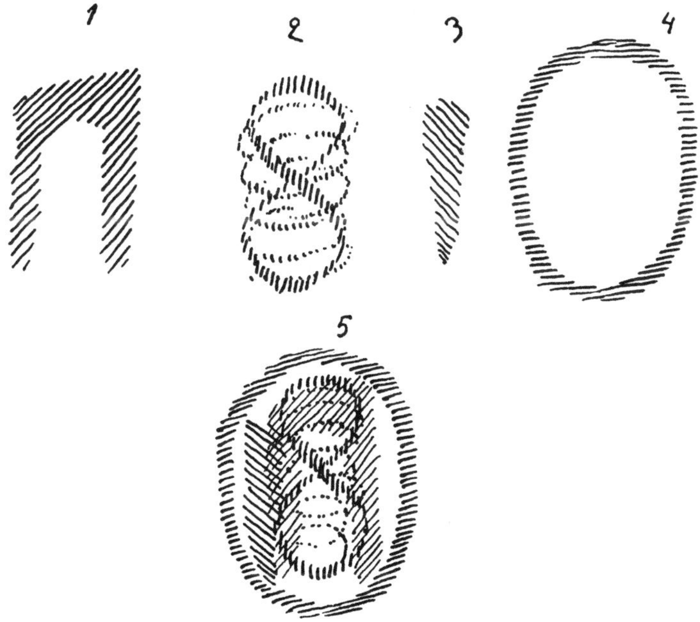

knowledge. However fanciful this may seem, it is the real human being shown, if I may put it like this, symbolically: the human being of paradise who does not consist of matter as he does today, but who has a truly supersensible nature.

What, then, became of the luciferic influence? Well, the luciferic influence caused the Imaginations to spray out through the bursting spirit; they sprayed into matter which became what we have today as our skeletal system. The skeletal system is the human being of Imagination filled in with matter. Matter is no part of the higher human being; it catapulted into what would have remained entirely with Imagination if the luciferic influence had not arrived. One would have been able to walk straight through a human being—which now sounds nonsensical—if these Imaginations had not first been drawn together and then additionally stuffed with bony matter. Now one would bump into the bones if one were to walk through the human being. He has become impermeable.

What came from the Spirits of Movement is filled out with muscular matter, and what would be perceptible as Intuition is filled out with nerve matter. And only now, in what goes beyond this, do we come to something supersensible, namely the human ether body which, although it is spiritual, does still contain the most tenuous matter, more tenuous even than nerve matter, and which is not in any way taken into consideration.

So you can see that the human being has become an exceedingly coarse creature. If he had become what the gods originally intended, he would have had no bones, and the supersensible bones of Imagination would have given him his form. He would have no muscles as instruments of movement; supersensible substance would have moved within him, whereas now what moves is everywhere spiked with muscular substance. That which the Spirits of Movement gave as supersensible movement has been transformed into the physical movement of the muscles; and that which the Spirits of Wisdom gave by way of Intuition has become in the sense-perceptible human being the nerve material spiked into the Intuition. And regarding the skeletal system depicted today in anatomy textbooks we can say: This was originally intended to be a pure Imagination but through the luciferic and the ahrimanic influence it has been so coarsened that we are now faced with these dense, thick, brittle, hard bones—so solidified have the Imaginations become.

Still, surely one can hardly say that no splendid reflection of Imagination can be found in the physical world! Those who know that this skeletal human being is an image of Imagination will certainly see the picture of the human skeleton as an image from the world of Imagination. And when you see a picture of the human muscular system you should really say to yourselves: This is entirely unnatural, inwardly it is a lie because I see it pictured instead of hearing it in spirit. This is because actually you are looking at supersensible rhythmical movement spiked with muscular matter, which should be removed. What remained would be invisible; it would be audible in the same way as the flowing movements of music are audible. Inspirations should really be audible. But what you see pictured as the muscular human being represents Inspirations spiked with matter. And as for the human being of nerves, you should neither see nor hear him but perceive him purely spiritually. For a cosmic view of the world such depictions are entirely out of place since what ought to be comprehended in pure spirituality is a spiritual wrapping spiked with physical matter, so that we are shown a visible depiction of what ought to be perceived solely as an Intuition.

This departure from paradise shows that the human being was indeed originally in the spiritual world, in paradise, where he consisted of Imagination, Inspiration and Intuition; in other words he was in an entirely unearthly existence. But then, through what he himself provoked through the luciferic influence, he became as though spiked with matter through what burst forth out of the spirit. This is what fills us but does not really belong to us. We bear this matter within us, and because we carry it in us we have to die physically. This is indeed the reason for physical death, and for much else also. Having as it were departed from his spiritual state, the human being is able to live here in physical existence only until matter overcomes what holds it together. The fact is that matter constantly wants to burst open, and the matter in the bones is only held together by the strength of Imagination. Once the strength of the bones gains the upper hand they are no longer capable of life. It is the same with the muscles and nerves. When the matter in bones, muscles and nerves gains the upper hand over Imagination, Inspiration and Intuition and can thus burst forth, then the human being has to lay aside his physical body. Herein, then, lies the connection between physical death and the luciferic influence. Tomorrow we shall investigate how evil and suchlike, illnesses and so on, came into the world.

LECTURE 5

HANOVER, 31 DECEMBER 1911

THE main purpose of yesterday's lecture was to gain insight into all the various complicated explanations concerning, initially, what we ought to regard as matter, as materiality. We saw matter, materiality, as burst spiritual forms, pulverized spiritual forms. In the context of these lectures it has been our task to point to the essential nature of physical existence from this angle because as human beings we are enveloped in this material existence. Bursting spiritual form has entered into us and filled us entirely. The expulsion from paradise is an apt symbolic depiction of this permeating of the human being with earthly matter.

If you followed what was being said yesterday not only in concepts but also by experiencing it to some extent, you will have reached a conception of how we, as human beings, are to some extent twofold beings. Consider what we said the day before yesterday about how the luciferic influence made it possible for the human being to have introduced into him the kind of sense perceptions we possess here in our earthly existence. We pointed out that these earthly sense perceptions were not initially intended for us since we should have had a way of living with the all-pervading will, and that the way we now hear through our ears, see through our eyes and perceive through our other sense-organs is in fact a deformity that has come about through the luciferic influence.

We also then, more within the human being, pointed out how secretions from the glands came about through a displacement of the members of the human organization. And finally we attributed the normal working of the organs, nutrition and all processing of substances within the human body, to a kind of preponderance of the astral body over the activity of the ether body, a preponderance which had also come about through the luciferic influence. This is what we arrived at the day before yesterday.

In other words, all the coarse material processes, the nutritional and digestive processes and so on, the processes of glandular secretion and also the processes of sense perception are, in the way they exist in us today, attributable to the influence of Lucifer. And yesterday we saw from another angle that we also owe to the luciferic influence the nerve material, the matter of which nerves are made; and the same applies to muscular matter and also bone matter.

Let us now look again at this twofold human being. On the one hand we owe sense perceptions, glandular activity and the whole organic process of metabolism to the luciferic influence; and on the other hand it is also to the luciferic influence that we owe the existence of the nerves, the muscular system and the bony system. So how do these two human beings behave, the being of the senses, glands and digestion on the one hand, and on the other hand the being of the nerves, the muscles and the bones? What is the cosmic, the universal task of these two in the way they are coupled together in human nature?

There is not even any need of spiritual insight in order to notice that everything connected with our senses, our glandular activity and our digestive system is, basically, transient or immediately perishable when it takes place within the human being. These are things which, by his very nature, the human being leaves behind him. It is obvious that there is no eternal purpose involved in our carrying out these organic activities. You need only examine briefly what science, or our daily life, teaches us before you say: As instruments of digestion and nourishment we are harnessed to life in a decidedly dreadful manner, for this is a wheel which turns forever in the same way. Unless you consider it great progress when someone, perhaps over years, develops preferences for new foods or drinks which he did not enjoy earlier on, you cannot help declaring: There is very little forward progress in this ever-churning treadmill of eating and digesting and so on. It is repeated over and over again in the same way, and hardly anyone will be likely even to dream that this activity gives us human beings any special value for eternity.

In the same way glandular secretion, too, has fulfilled its purpose as soon as it has taken place. Of course it is important for the organism as a whole, but it certainly has no value for eternity. And since sense impressions come and go, the same also applies to perception by means of the senses. You need only consider how pale, even after just a few days, a sense impression has become, how much it differs from the memory of the sense perception you experienced—how very different the memory is from the sense perception—and you will not fail to realize that however beautiful sensory perceptions are, however much pleasure your observation of them provides, they have no value for eternity. Where is the value which arose out of the sense impressions you had as a child or a young person? Where is it all, whatever it was that approached you through eyes or ears? How pale are those memories!

When you consider that in so far as he is a creature of glands and digestion the human being gains no value for eternity through these activities, when you consider this you will now find it easy to connect this thought with the general description we gave yesterday—because unfortunately only brief hints can be given in short lectures—namely the idea of the bursting, shattering form. As form spurts into these activities, thus, so to speak, providing the organism with collapsing form—that is, with matter—it does so in such a way that the activity of the senses, the secretion of the glands and the activity of digestion comes about. And this shows us vividly that here we are confronted with form which is breaking up, form which is shattering into pieces. In the activity of the senses, in the secretion of the glands and in the activity of digestion we are presented with specific processes of the disintegration of form. These are specific processes within whatever we describe in general as the process of the disintegration of form or as the spurting of form into matter.

If we now turn to nerve activity, to muscle activity and to the working of the bones, the existence of the bones in the human being, we are confronted with an entirely different situation. Yesterday we mentioned that the bony system in a way contains Imagination brought into matter, that the muscular system in its movement contains Inspiration brought into matter, and that the nervous system contains Intuition brought into matter.

We now come to something that has been discussed only approximately in more general lectures on spiritual science, and that is the way in which, when the human being passes through the portal of death, his bony system disintegrates, whether through decomposition, through cremation or by any other means. But what remains when the bony system disintegrates physically is Imagination; the Imagination is not lost. It remains in those substances which we also have within us when we have passed through the portal of death and are entering into kamaloka or devachan. We retain an image-configuration, although when this is viewed by a thoroughly schooled clairvoyant it does not very much resemble our skeleton. But when a less highly trained clairvoyant allows this to work on him he does see in this image-configuration an outward resemblance to the human bony system, which is why it is not so wrong to depict death in the image of a skeleton even though this derives from an unschooled yet not entirely inappropriate clairvoyance.

Also included in Imagination is what is left of the muscles once they have disintegrated physically. Inspiration remains, of which the muscles are merely an expression because they are really only Inspirations permeated with materiality. So we retain Inspiration when we have passed through the portal of death. This is very interesting. And we also retain an Intuition of the nervous system when the nerves themselves are approaching their disintegration after death. All these aspects are true constituents of our astral and our ether bodies.

As you know, we do not entirely discard our ether body for we carry an extract of the ether body with us after having passed through the portal of death. And this is not all. As we go on our way through the world we carry our nervous system with us, and this nervous system is nothing other than Intuition permeated with matter. As we carry this nervous system about with us there is, at those points where the nerves are interspersed throughout our body, a continuous presence of Intuition, and from this Intuition spirituality streams forth which permanently surrounds us like an aura. So as we pass through the portal of death it is not only a matter of what we take with us, for there is in addition also this Intuition which streams forth in proportion to the disintegration of the nerves. There is within us a permanent process of disintegration; we are constantly in need of reconstruction, whereby the durability is greatest in the case of the nervous system; and there is a constant streaming out which can only be perceived through Intuition.

We can therefore say: Substance that can be perceived through Intuition, spiritual substance, constantly streams forth from the human being in the same measure as his physical nervous system disintegrates. So we can see that as he makes use of his physical nervous system, wearing it out, causing it to disintegrate, the human being is not without significance for the world. Indeed, he is very significant for it, since the substances perceptible to Intuition which stream forth from him depend on the uses to which he puts his nerves. And similarly, as the human being makes use of his muscles, substances perceptible to Inspiration stream forth from him. And that which beams forth in this way constantly populates the world with all kinds of exceedingly differentiated movement processes. Thus substances stream forth that are perceptible to Inspiration—this way of expressing it is inadequate, but we have no other. And from the bones of the human being substance streams forth that can be perceived through Imagination.

This, now, is especially interesting. I do not want to overfeed you with the results of clairvoyant research, but this is truly interesting, namely that through the raying out from the bones as they disintegrate, the human being everywhere leaves behind him, as it were, images, spiritual pictures perceptible to Imagination; delicate shadow pictures are left behind by us wherever we have been. As you depart from this hall you will leave behind you on the seats delicate shadow images which for a while will remain perceptible to a more subtle, well-trained clairvoyance until the general processes of the universe absorb them. Delicate shadow images, which have streamed forth from your skeletal system, will be left behind by each one of you.

It is such Imaginations which bring about those uncomfortable inklings we sometimes experience upon entering a room where someone else, some disagreeable person, has been. This is mainly due to the Imaginations he has left behind. We still find him there in a kind of shadow image. A sufficiently sensitive person is no less capable in this respect than a clairvoyant, for he senses the unpleasantness left behind in a room by someone else. The clairvoyant merely has the added ability to describe what the sensitive person only surmises.

What, then, becomes of everything that radiates from us? Taken all in all, dear friends, we can say that there are emanations from everything we do in the world. Whenever you are doing something or going around you are bringing your system of bones and muscles into movement. Indeed, even while you are lying down and thinking about something you radiate substance that can be detected through Intuition. In short, with every activity you constantly send something out into the world.

If these processes did not take place there would be nothing left of the earth once it reached its goal apart from pulverized matter, which would pass over into the rest of the universe in the form of dust. But whatever human beings rescue out of the material processes of the earth continues to live on in the general cosmos, in the universal world, in all that comes into being through Intuition, Inspiration and Imagination. Thus human beings give back to the world the building bricks needed for rebuilding itself. All this will live on as the spirit and soul of the whole earth once its material aspect disintegrates like a corpse in the same way as individual human souls live on in spirit once the individual has passed through the portal of death. The human being conveys his own soul through the portal of death; and the earth conveys across to the Jupiter existence all that has arisen out of the Intuitions, Inspirations and Imaginations of human beings.

In this way we have characterized the great difference between the one part and the other part of the human being in so far as he is a twofold being. The part which grasps hold of sense perceptions, which secretes through glands, and which digests and nourishes itself—this is the human being destined to bring about all that is cleft and riven in the temporal realm. But whatever is developed through the existence of the nervous, muscular and bony systems is incorporated into the earth so that it may be enabled to continue in existence.

We are now approaching a mystery which is a part of our overall existence, and being a mystery it cannot really be grasped by our intellect. It needs to be believed and penetrated, and it is nonetheless true. That which human beings are capable of sending out into their surroundings is clearly composed of a duality. There is one part of Inspiration, Intuition and Imagination upon which general cosmic existence depends and which it absorbs; general cosmic existence accepts this part, but there is another part which it does not accept, which it rejects. The general cosmos declares: Yes, I can do with these Inspirations, Intuitions and Imaginations; these I can accept in order to carry them over into the Jupiter existence. But others are rejected by it, it does not accept them. And as a result those Intuitions, Inspirations and Imaginations are not accepted anywhere and thus come to a halt. They remain spiritually within the cosmos and cannot be absorbed. Thus, what rays out from us falls into two parts, into one part which the cosmos is glad to accept and another which it rejects, which it finds unacceptable and does not take up. This latter part is left standing.

How long does it remain standing? It remains standing there until the human being comes and destroys it himself by means of emitting what is capable of destroying it. And as a rule only the one who has created it is capable of emitting what will destroy it. Here we have the practicality of karma; here we have the reason why we are obliged to encounter once again during the course of our karma all those Imaginations, Inspirations and Intuitions that have been rejected by the cosmos. It is up to us to destroy them, because the cosmos only accepts what is correct in thinking, beautiful in feeling and good in morality. It rejects everything else. That is the mystery. And whatever is wrong in thinking, ugly in feeling and bad or evil in morality must be expunged from existence by the human being himself through thoughts, feelings and impulses of will, or by deeds, if it is not to continue to exist. Such things will pursue him until he manages to expunge them.

We have thus reached the point where we are shown how untrue it is that the cosmos consists only of neutral laws of nature or expresses itself only through neutral laws of nature. The cosmos all around us, which we believe ourselves capable of comprehending through our senses and our intellect, possesses quite other forces. It is, we could say, a stern repudiator of what is evil, ugly or false, and it is keen to take in the good, the beautiful and the true. The powers that be in the cosmos do not sit in judgement only at certain times. Sitting in judgement is something they do constantly, throughout the whole of earthly evolution.

We are now able to answer the question: What is the overall situation with regard to the development of the human being in relation to the higher spiritual beings?

We have seen that on the one hand the human being of the senses, the glands and the digestion can be said to have arisen through the luciferic influence. But to some extent we can also attribute the other human being to that same luciferic influence. Whereas the former is the human being of deterioration destined only for temporal existence, the latter has the task of saving what is human for eternity, for all duration, taking it across to a later existence. It is the task of the man of nerves, muscles and bones to carry across what human beings experience on the earth. We conclude from this basically that man has fallen from spiritual heights through having become the first type, the human being of senses, glands and digestion, and that he will gradually be enabled to work his way up again into spiritual existence through having received the counterbalance of nerves, muscles and bones.

The strange thing, however, is that this separating out of Intuitive, Inspired and Imaginative substance can only take place because the processes of matter represent destructive processes. If our nerves, if our muscles, if our bones were not constantly deteriorating, if they were to remain as they are, then we would be unable to separate this off, for it is only through deterioration on the one side, as expressed in material existence, that the flashing up, the lighting up of the spirit can come about. If our nerves, our muscles and our bones were unable to deteriorate and finally fall prey to death, then we would be condemned to exist only within the earth as it is, without being able to participate in further development towards the future. We would participate in a rigid, petrified present time lacking any development towards a future. The forces that play their part both in the one kind and in the other kind of human existence are indeed two forces that balance one another out.

And between the two, as though mediating between them, we have that substance, that form of matter, about which we have spoken more often in connection with general aspects of spiritual science but less often in the present context. It is blood which mediates between the two, and which is, also in this context, 'a juice of rarest quality'.[24] We have seen that as far as the substance of the nerves and so on is concerned it has come to work in the way it does through the luciferic influence. But with the blood the situation is that the very substance itself is what fell prey to the luciferic influence. As we saw, the way in which physical body, ether body and astral body collaborate with one another would have been different if no luciferic influence had occurred. In these cases there are certain supersensible aspects which take up the physical matter and only then, through the luciferic influence, make it what it has become. Nerve, muscle and bone substances come into being as a result of certain bodies in the human being not combining together in the right way. Lucifer has no influence on the substances as such because these substances do not arise until he has, as it were, brought the arrangement of the bodies into disorder. Wherever Lucifer has approached the human being he has brought about this disorder.

But his influence on the blood—on the matter, the very substance of the blood itself—has been direct. Blood is 'a juice of rarest quality' because it is the only physical substance which as such manifests that in its very nature it is not as it ought to have been in the human being of today if there had been no luciferic interference. Blood has become something entirely different from what it should have been. This is grotesque, is it not, but it is so.

Let us remind ourselves of how matter came into being. We said that matter arises when spiritual form reaches a certain boundary and then shatters, so that this pulverized form represents matter. This earthly matter shows itself like this only in its mineral form since the other substances are changed in other ways. Blood is the exceptional substance.

Originally blood as a substance was also intended to reach down to a specific boundary of form. Here (a, *see opposite*) you see the purely spiritual form-rays of the blood, and here (b) its strength would have been exhausted. But according to its original tendency the blood was not supposed to spray out into space. Here (b) at the boundary it was to have become just a little bit like matter before spraying back into itself (the dots going upwards), before spraying directly back into the

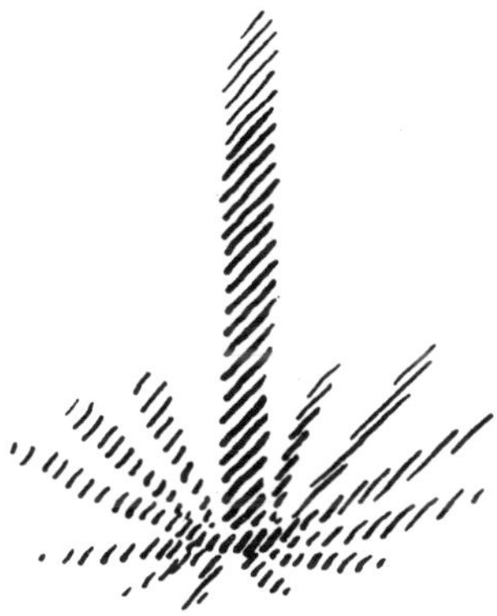

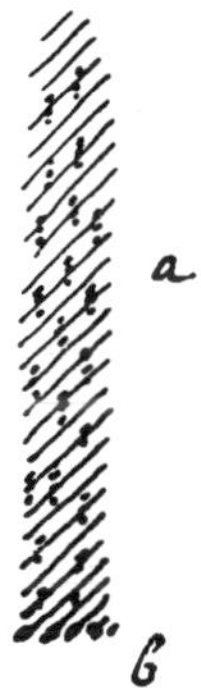

spiritual. This is how blood was originally intended to be. If I may put it more bluntly, blood would have reached only as far as forming a thin skin where matter begins so that it would emerge from the spiritual only momentarily, becoming only slightly physically perceptible before darting back into the spiritual and being received there by the spiritual realm. Blood was intended to become like a continual flowing out and darting back into the spiritual.

This is the predisposition of blood. It should have been a continual lighting up into matter while remaining entirely spiritual. This is what it would have become if at the beginning of earthly evolution human beings had received their 'I' solely from the Spirits of Form. They would then have sensed their 'I' by the resistance which this momentary shining out in the blood signifies. In this shining out in the blood the human being would have sensed the 'I am', and this would have been the organ for perceiving his 'I'. It would have been his sole sensory perception since the others would not have come about if everything had run its course without the luciferic influence. This would have amounted to living with the all-pervading will. What had been intended for the human being was that his one sensory perception should have consisted in perceiving his 'I' in the shining out of the blood substance and its immediate darting back into the spiritual. The intention was that instead of seeing colours, hearing sounds, experiencing tastes, the human being would live in the all-pervading will. It should have been like floating in the all-pervading will.

What was intended for him was that, having been placed into the spiritual world as pure Imagination, Inspiration and Intuition, he would look down from there at a being on the earth or in its vicinity. But he would not feel: I am enclosed within that being. Instead he would feel: I look down and perceive something which belongs to me; the one and only thing of matter shines out to me, that which is spiritual blood becoming matter; it is in this that I perceive my 'I'.

The only perception to be experienced through the senses should have been the perception of the 'I', and the only substance intended for the human being in the realm of matter would have been blood in the form of that momentary shining forth. If this is what the human being would have become by remaining the human being of paradise looking down out of the universe upon what had been intended to symbolize him on this earth, then a purely spiritual being consisting of Imaginations, Inspirations and Intuitions would have experienced the momentary shining out of the blood as his 'I'. In that momentary shining forth the human being would then have been able to say: I am, for down there I am bringing into being something which is a part of me.

It is remarkable that we can really say: Actually, the human being was destined to live in the environs of the earth. A human being living here in the environs of the earth (a) was to have created his own mirror image (b) on the earth in order through that momentary shining forth to beam back his 'I' and say: Down there is the manifestation of me. It

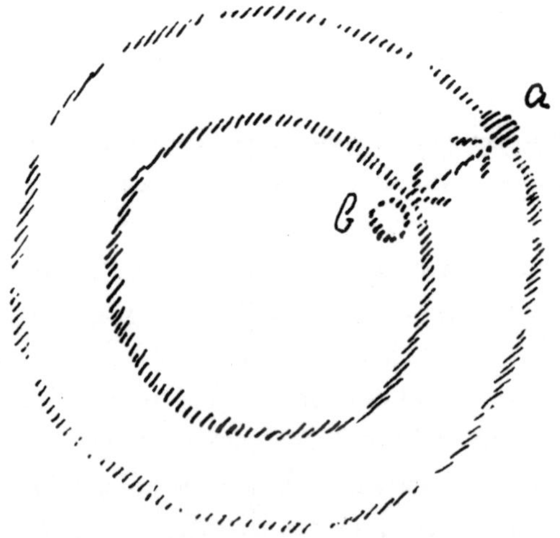

was not supposed to be the case that the human being has to carry around with him his man of bones, muscles and nerves, his man of glands; nor should it have been necessary constantly to form the grotesque judgement: This is what I am. Something different should have come about. The human being should have lived in the environs of the earthly planet, engraving his sign upon the earth through the shining out of the blood form, saying: Here I drive in my stake, my seal and my sign which gives me awareness of my 'I'. With what I have become through the Saturn, through the Sun and through the Moon existences I float out here in the universal all. All I need then do is add the 'I' which I perceive as I inscribe myself down there; then I can always read that which I am in the shining forth of the blood. Yes indeed, it was not originally intended that we should walk about in bodies made of bones and flesh as we do. We should have been circling the earth while making signs down there through which to recognize that this is who we are, that what we are is an 'I'. Those who do not take this into account cannot know the being of man.

Lucifer then came and brought it about that the human being should not only know his 'I' as a sense perception but should also experience as his 'I' everything he had already possessed on Moon as his astral body: thinking, feeling and will. His 'I' was mixed together with these. But this made it necessary for the human being to descend into matter. The first consequence of this was the change in the blood which then no longer shone out for a moment before being taken back into spirituality. Instead the substance of the blood pressed in and burst forth; it became something which bursts forth and shatters. Thus the substance of the blood, which ought to return to the spiritual realm as soon as it becomes material, now spurts out into the rest of the human being, filling his whole organization and becoming transformed in compliance with the forces in that organization. Depending on whether it penetrates into a preponderance, let's say, of the physical body over the ether body, or of the ether body over the astral body, and so on, it turns into the substance of nerves, the substance of muscles and so on. In this way Lucifer forced the blood into a coarser substantiality. Whereas blood was intended to shine forth briefly as matter and then immediately disappear again, Lucifer forced it to enter into coarser materiality.

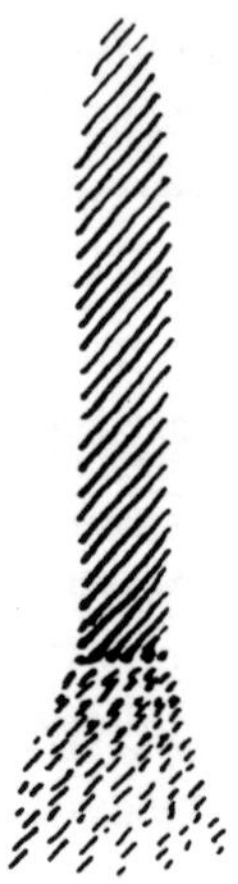

This is the direct achievement of Lucifer: transforming blood into matter. At least with the other members he only brought about disorder. Blood would not exist at all in the way it does now; it would in its spirituality only come close to the border with matter, *in statu nascendi*, before immediately pulling back again. In its present material form blood is a luciferic creation. And because the human being now has the physical expression of his 'I' in his blood, this human being is, here on earth, linked through his 'I' with Lucifer's creation.

And since, moreover, it became possible for Ahriman to approach the human being after Lucifer had been there first, we can say: Lucifer threw down the blood so that Ahriman could catch it; so now both of them are able to lay hold of the human being. Need we be surprised that according to an age-old tradition Lucifer-Ahriman regards blood as his own earthly possession? Is it surprising that he expects contracts to be signed in blood, that he coerces Faust into signing the contract with him in his own blood?[25] Blood is out and out his very own by right! Everything else contains some element of the divine and makes him feel uncomfortable. For Lucifer even ink is more divine than blood which is his very own element.

We have seen that the human being consists of two parts: the man of senses, glands and digestion, and the man of nerves, muscles and bones. In their coarse materiality both these parts are supplied with suitable forces by what blood has become through the luciferic influence. Even from external science we can learn that in so far as he is a physical being man is entirely the outcome of his blood. All physical matter in the human being is nourished by his blood; he is transformed blood. In so far as they consist of physical matter, the bones, nerves, muscles, glands, indeed all the parts are transformed blood. Actually the human being is blood, and in so far as he is blood he is the living Lucifer-Ahriman himself; he carries Lucifer with him all the time. Only in what he has within him which is beyond what the blood has given him does the human being also belong to the divine worlds, to on-going evolution which does not remain retarded. Lucifer came into the world through having become backward at a certain level of development, and the same goes for Ahriman.

When we examine what has just been described we shall be able to say: From the beginning of earthly evolution human beings possessed something which they shared. They had something very much in common in their blood, namely if this blood had remained for them what had been intended from the outset then it would have been a pure emanation from the Spirits of Form. The Spirits of Form would have existed in our blood as it originally was. As most of you know, these Spirits of Form are none other than the seven Elohim of the Bible. You need only leaf through the lectures I gave on Genesis in Munich[26] and you will discover that—if he had retained his blood in the form originally intended—the human being would feel the seven Elohim within him. That is, he would sense his 'I' to be sevenfold, with the main member corresponding for him with Yahweh or Jehovah and the other six initially being subsidiary members. If the human being's blood had not been spoilt by Lucifer, this sevenfold entity, which he would sense as being his 'I' or the seven Elohim or Spirits of Form, would have taught him something which we are now, with much effort, obliged to regain as knowledge of the sevenfold nature of the human being.

This is how long humanity—on account of that damaged blood—has had to wait before being able to recognize that a sevenfoldness is involved. This is how long that damaged blood has made us wait before we can become mature enough—thanks to sufficient emanations of Intuitive, Inspirative and Imaginative substance coming from nerves, muscles and bones—to regain that sevenfoldness of our human nature!

Now we can specify, initially in an abstract form, that nature of the human being which is brought into play in the 'I' by the physical body and by the ether body, that nature which is brought into play by the astral body, from itself—Yahweh or Jehovah—and also that part which is brought into play by the Manas or Spirit Self, that part which is brought into play by the Buddhi or Life Spirit, and that part which is brought into play by the Atma or Spirit Man. But the human being would not have reached a specific darkening of the other six members, and a special brightening of the one member, the 'I', if Lucifer had not been sent in during the course of earthly evolution. At the beginning of earthly evolution the other members became darkened while the 'I' became bright, shining out in its brighter 'I'-ishness. This occurred because in the material sense this 'I' was forced into dense matter so that it should gain a thorough awareness of being a unity, a singularity, after having initially felt itself to be sevenfold.

So we see that, if his blood had remained in its original state, the human being would have attained an 'I' which possessed a sevenfold character from the beginning. But because of Lucifer becoming involved he attained an 'I' with the characteristic of uniqueness so that he came to feel and know his 'I' as the very centre of his being. Since the seven Elohim were originally intended to manifest in every human 'I', we can now comprehend the blood as something that was originally intended to bring human beings together, to enable them to form a social whole and thus feel themselves as the all-embracing human species. It is due to what Lucifer gave to human beings that they regard themselves as an individual 'I', as a specific individual who in his independence is recognizable as being distinct from the overall human species. This shows us that in the universal development of the earth the human being is coming to be led by Lucifer to be increasingly independent, whereas through the seven Elohim he would increasingly come to feel himself as a member of overall humanity. What this implies for morality and the development of human life as a whole will be our subject for tomorrow.

Lecture 6

HANOVER, 1 JANUARY 1912

You may have gathered especially from these lectures how very complicated the human being is and from how many angles he has to be considered if we want to come to grips with truly understanding him. For the moment we now have one more fact to bring forward, one of the most important facts about the human being's development if we intend to consider through clairvoyant research both the path of his evolution in ages long past and also the future prospects of the human species.

During the course of these lectures I have told you about how we can educate our capacity for knowledge and our desire for knowledge through absorbing the conditions of soul which we termed amazement, reverence, wisdom-filled harmony with the world's phenomena and acquiescence towards all the happenings in the universe, and how in doing this we can gradually advance our knowledge to the point where we can, in everything we have around us, distinguish between on the one hand something which is coming into being and will only attain its completion in the future and, on the other hand, something which is slowly dwindling away and vanishing. It is in the realm of coming into being and dying away that we perceive these things.

I pointed out specifically that the human larynx is actually an organ of the future and that it is intended to be something entirely different from what it is today. Today it merely tells the outer world, by means of the spoken word, what is going on in our inner being. But in the future it will communicate everything we ourselves are; in other words, it will serve to bring the whole human being into the world. It will be the future organ of reproduction. In future the human being will not merely express to the world, through the word and with the help of the larynx, what is going on in his inner being; he will give to the world an expression of himself as a totality: human reproduction will be dependent on the organ of the larynx.

In this complicated microcosm, in this complicated miniature world known as the human being, for every organ which is at present in the phase of being a seed, and which will in the future attain a higher degree of perfection, there is another organ which is, shall we say, in a process of gradual diminishment and dying away. In the case of the human larynx the corresponding organ of decline is the organ of hearing. In whatever degree the hearing of the human being increasingly disappears, declining more and more, in the same degree the larynx will become an organ of ever greater perfection and ever greater significance.

We can only comprehend the immense importance of this fact by going with the help of the Akashic Record into a far-distant past of humanity. Out of what we are able to discover there, we shall then build a picture of what the organ of hearing, the ear, originally was. With regard to knowledge about the human being it is immensely enlightening to follow the ear into the past. As it is today the human ear truly is a mere shadow of what it used to be. Today it can hear only sounds or the words of the physical plane as they are expressed through sounds. This is the final remnant of what used to flow into the human being through his hearing. It is the last remnant, for once upon a time there flowed into the human being through his hearing all the mighty movements of the whole universe. Today we hear only earthly music through our ears, but in those ancient times what the human being heard was the music of the universe, the music of the spheres. And just as today we clothe words in the sounds of music so, long ago, were the divine words of God clothed in the music of the spheres, those words which the Gospel of John proclaims as the divine universal word, the Logos. It was the heavenly music, the music of the spheres, which flowed into everything we can describe as the hearing of the distant past in the same way as today only human words and earthly music flow. And within that music of the spheres were the words spoken by the divine spirits. Just as today people form the air with their words and with their song, so did the divine music bring forth forms.

And the most precious of these forms can come before our souls as follows. Think of speaking a word today, or perhaps simply a vowel such as 'ah'. And think of how, when this 'ah' enters into the air, the possibility arises of creating a form within this air. This is how forms came forth into the world from the Logos, and the most precious of all those forms is the human being. In his primordial form the human being was generated by being spoken out of the cosmic word. The gods spoke, and just as, today, forms enter into the air through human speaking, so did our world enter into its forms through the word of the gods. And the most precious of all those forms is the human being.

Of course in those times the organ of hearing was as yet far, far more complicated. Since then it has shrunk. What we possess today as our external organ of hearing, which only penetrates a little way into the brain, then came in from the outside and extended across the whole human being. And within the human being as a whole the surging of the waves spread out, speaking the human being out of the divine word and into the world. Thus was the human being spiritually created through the organ of hearing. And in the future, when he has risen up again, the human being will possess only a rudimentary ear, a completely shrunken ear. The purpose of the ear will be entirely a thing of the past.

The ear is in decline. But in its place the larynx, now still a seed, will have developed to higher glory and greater perfection. In its perfection it will utter that which the human being is capable of bringing forth for the world as a reiteration of his being, just as once the gods uttered the human being as their creation, speaking him forth into the earth.

In this way the forward march of the world is, in a way, turned back. The whole human being about whom we have been speaking is, as he stands before us, the product of a descending development; and when we look at an organ such as his ear we have to say: This ear which has become so dense in its boniness right down to those inner ossicles, this ear is as it were the final stage of a descending development. The sense-perceptible as such disappears, but the human being develops forwards into the world of spirituality, and his ascending organs are the bridges which lead him upwards to the spirit. Thus the world of the senses relates to the world of the spirit in that the world of the senses is shown to us as a whole collection of expiring organs while the world of the spirit can be seen through organs in the process of creation.

And this is also taking place in what we can perceive of the world. There is everywhere a process of coming into being and passing away again, and much can be learned from this idea of coming into being and dying away. It is important and meaningful to apply it to the rest of the world. Thus there is in the mineral realm, for example, something which is undergoing a process of ascending development, being at present in a kind of seed condition. And that is mercury, quicksilver. Quicksilver is a metal which will undergo transformations, changes towards a more perfect state. Quicksilver has as yet not pulverized all those forces which substances possess in their spiritual state before becoming matter. It will in future be able to put forth additional important aspects of its spirituality and adopt different forms so that in the mineral realm it will in certain ways correspond with the human larynx and also in certain ways with the organ to which the larynx is attached: the lungs. Other metals, such as copper for example, are instead now in a kind of descending development. In future this will become evident as follows: Copper will no longer possess inner spiritual forces which it can put forth; instead it will increasingly merely splinter and decay, becoming cosmic dust.

Other correlations like those just mentioned as examples will from now on come to be increasingly investigated. People will increasingly study the relationship between coming into being and dying away in the different realms of nature. They will come to realize, not only by experimentation but through Imagination, that they can find specific relationships of metallic substances with specific organs of the human body. They will then also realize through Imagination how these substances—whose effectiveness is partially also known through external experience—can in addition have healing effects for the human body through their regenerative and restorative powers. Indeed the relationships of the various realities will come to light in all kinds of ways.[27]

In the case of plants, people will come to realize that whatever exists in the seed, in the power of the seed, is related to the human being in ways different from how the forces in the roots, for example, relate to him. Whatever is contained in the roots of the plant corresponds in a certain way with the human brain and the related nervous system (see chart on p. 82). This is the case to such an extent that in fact whatever is contained in the roots we eat has a bearing on the processes that occur in the brain and the nervous system. So if a person wants, as it were, to exert a physical influence on his brain and nervous system as physical tools of a spiritual life, then he will take in with his food the forces that are contained in the roots of plants. He will in a way allow what he takes in as food to do the thinking or the spiritual work within him. On the other hand, if he is less inclined to absorb the root-nature, then in his own spirituality he will himself be the one who makes use of his brain and nervous system. This shows that eating a great deal of root-food prevents the human being from becoming independent in his soul and spiritual experiences; the objective, external realm is working through him, owing to the way in which his brain and his nervous system have become separated off. So if we want chiefly our own self to work within us, then we must exercise restraint with regard to the amount of root-food we consume.

My dear friends, these remarks are not intended in any way as instructions about following some kind of diet but merely as information regarding certain facts of nature. I must warn strongly against following any such rules without further ado. Not every individual has reached the stage at which he can cope with letting what is objective take over his power of thinking. It can very easily happen that, when an insufficiently mature individual allows the power of his thinking and feeling to be taken over by an objective soul life, then, having avoided eating root-foods from the realm of plants, he will enter into a state of sleepiness. This is because his spiritual and soul component is not yet strong enough to develop within itself the powers of the spirit which would otherwise develop objectively within him without the help of the spirit and soul component. This is the situation. Any diet a person might choose to follow is an entirely individual matter which is very much bound up with how he has developed in one way or another.

What is contained in plant leaves, for example, is related to what we regard as the lungs, as the whole system of the lungs. We can draw something like a balance-sheet in a person. For example, if someone has a respiratory system which has developed more from within, perhaps through heredity or for some other reason, then it would be good to advise him not to eat too much food involving plant leaves. But another person might be better advised to help his respiratory system by eating a great many foods containing leaves. Such things are connected with the powers of healing out there in the world, in the different realms of nature. The various parts of the plant relating to the different organs are those which contain healing forces for those various organs in the human organism. Thus plant roots contain many healing forces in relation to the nervous system. Leaves contain many healing forces in relation to the lungs. The flowers of a plant contain many healing forces in relation to the system of the kidneys, for example. And plant seeds contain, in a sense, healing forces in relation to the heart; the forces of seeds provide healing in relation to the heart, but only in cases where the heart opposes the circulation of the blood too strongly. If the heart gives in too readily to the blood circulation, then it is preferably the fruits, the seeds which have fully ripened into fruits, which may be considered.

Roots	—	Brain
Leaves	—	Lungs
Flowers	—	Kidneys
Seeds	—	Heart
Fruits	—	Blood system

These are specific hints which arise when we look outwards from the human being and observe nature all around us. What appears to our senses in this surrounding nature, what belongs to the world of the senses, is in fact merely superficial. The part of plants that belongs to the sense-perceptible world is purely superficial; behind the part of the plant that is perceived by our eyes, our sense of taste, our sense of smell lie its spiritual and soul forces. But these spiritual and soul forces of the plant are not contained within it in such a way that we can speak of every plant having a soul of its own as we can speak of every individual human being possessing a soul. That is not the case. Someone who believes that every plant has its own soul makes the same mistake as thinking that a human being's every hair, or an earlobe, or his nose or a tooth possesses a soul.

It is the whole human being who possesses a soul, and we can only gain some insight into the human being when we see all his parts as a single whole. We must do this with regard to every being. With every being we must take care to note whether it is a part or whether it is a totality. Wherever they are on the earth, plants cannot be taken to form a totality; they are parts, members, and we only speak of a reality when we speak of whatever it is to which the plants belong as its parts, as its members. In the human being we can see this physically, we can see the whole, of which his teeth, his earlobe, his fingers are parts. We see the totality of his organism physically. In the case of the plants we do not see with our physical eyes the totality of which they are parts; we do not perceive this with a physical organ. Here we move directly from the part to the whole, we enter directly into the spiritual. Here what we have to say is: It is the soul element of the plant world which possesses the plants as its organs. There are very few beings in the totality of our earth, beings which are as though stuffed together in the earth and which possess separate parts such as plants in the way the human being possesses the hairs on his head.

When we want to go beyond plants in so far as they are visible to our senses, then we come to the group souls of the plants; these are the totality of which plants are the parts. Overall there are seven group souls which belong to the earth as plant souls; and for them the centre of the earth is, in a sense, the centre of their being. Thus we can think of the earth as more than merely a physical ball, for it is permeated by seven such larger or smaller spheres all of which have something like their own spiritual centre in the centre of the earth. And these spiritual beings then push the plants upwards out of the earth. The root grows downwards towards the centre of the earth; that is where it wishes to go, but it is prevented from reaching the centre by the physical material of the earth. Every plant root is striving to penetrate down to the centre of the earth, where the centre of the spiritual being to which the plant belongs is situated.

So now we see how extraordinarily important is the principle which tells us that we must always go towards the whole, and that with every living thing we must observe whether it is a part or a totality. In more recent times some researchers have come to regard plants as possessing souls; they see each individual plant as having its own soul.[28] This is no more clever than calling a tooth a human being, which amounts to a similar kind of jest. When researchers today talk of plants having souls, many people think this sounds almost anthroposophical, yet it is no more than scientific nonsense and should be pulped. Looking for individual souls in plants is akin to extracting a person's tooth and then searching for a human soul inside it. The plant soul cannot be found in individual plants. The most important part of the plant soul lies at the centre of the earth; and it is this, the most spiritual part of plant existence, which the root is striving to reach.

To examine a realm of this kind is, as far as modern science is concerned, an endeavour to examine the very portal of truth in the way Mephistopheles leads Faust towards the realm of the Mothers, towards the very portal but not right into the realm of the Mothers.[29] For just as Mephistopheles is unable to lead Faust right down into the realm of the Mothers, so is modern science also unable to enter fully into the realm of the spirit. Yet just as Mephistopheles provides the key, so does modern science provide the key. But science does not want to enter the realm of the spirit, and neither does Mephistopheles want to enter the realm of the Mothers. What science does is give us clues, and if we recognize these in what I have been describing in these lectures, then this recognition will often lead us to the portal of truth.

This is how modern science expresses itself in the words of Darwin when endeavouring to arrive at an important scientific principle merely through what the senses reveal, namely the principle of the so-called 'struggle for life'.[30] How can we fail to notice this struggle for life everywhere if we pay attention only to what the external world of the senses shows us? We are everywhere confronted with this struggle for life! See how much spawn, how many germs are cast into the ocean or onto the sand by the creatures of the sea, and how many of these perish and how few grow into adult creatures; how little of the spawn develops into animals and how much comes to nothing. In this alone we observe a seemingly frightful struggle for life and might be drawn into lamentation if we took only the sense-perceptible world into account: How many of these millions upon millions of germs perish in the struggle for life, and how few of them escape.

But this is only one aspect of the thought, and you can also begin at the other end of it. In order to guide your thinking towards a specific direction I would ask you to take hold of the thought at the other end. For you could turn your attention instead to a field of wheat with all those many ears bearing all those many wheat grains, and once again begin to lament about the struggle for life. How many of those grains of wheat will be lost as far as their ultimate aim is concerned? And how many of them will be planted once more into the earth in order to be renewed again as was the case with the old ones? We survey the field of wheat as it buds and sprouts with all its sumptuous fruitfulness and say: So much of all that budding and sprouting will come to nothing without having fulfilled its purpose and so little will be planted in the earth again so that new plants of the same kind may come into being. So here, too, in a somewhat different sphere, it is the same as in the case of the sea creatures where so little of what they produce comes to fruition.

A different question now arises: What would become of the human beings who need food to eat if all the grains of wheat were to be put back into the earth. Imagine all the grains of wheat producing plants once more. What would then become of all those creatures who gain their nourishment from the grains of wheat! It is worth taking note of how this overturns a belief which might appear justified when applied solely to the sense-perceptible world. It might seem justifiable in respect of the purely sense-perceptible field of wheat if we were to expect every grain to become a whole new plant. But perhaps this is an erroneous point of view. Perhaps in the world as a whole it is incorrect to think that every grain of wheat has the purpose of becoming a new plant. Perhaps there is nothing to justify the view that those grains which serve as food for other creatures have failed in their ultimate purpose, just as there is no reason to believe that the spawn, the germs of the sea creatures have failed in their purpose if they do not again become fish.

It really is nothing but a human presumption to claim that every seed must again produce another creature of the same kind. We can only correctly gauge the task of individual beings if we take account of the whole. When the seeds of the ocean perish in their millions without becoming fish once again, they are serving other creatures as food, they are sacrificing themselves for the sake of others. It is surely true that those spiritual substances which fight their way into existence in the seemingly perishing germs of the ocean do not lament about failing to attain their purpose when they become food for other creatures. We human beings remove ourselves with our intellect and look at everything from the outside. It is we who believe that there is meaning only in whatever strives to attain what we consider to be the aim as seen through our senses. An unprejudiced view of nature regards every stage of every creature as being complete. This completeness rests not in what a creature will become but in what it is.

These are the considerations arising from spiritual research which must be suggested to you. If you now turn away from the outer world and look into your soul, you will find it filled with thoughts which constantly flow into it and come to life there although only few of them are clearly grasped; only a few of these thoughts come to be a conscious part of the human soul. Go for a walk somewhere in the town and note how many impressions enter into your soul through your senses and yet how little of all this you observe in a way that will become an integral part of your soul life. You continuously absorb impressions, but the proportion of these impressions that become permanently resident in your soul reminds us of the proportion of the huge mass of annual fish spawnings that become fully-developed fish.

In the foundations of your inner soul life there is a wide expanse where you continuously have to select the little which can come to fruition. If we become aware even only partially of the oceanic flood of fanciful images and notions from which we emerge upon awakening from sleep, perhaps with dreams still showing last vestiges of the immensely fertile life we lead when asleep, then we may come to realize the significance of having absorbed so very much which cannot enter fully into our consciousness. The fact is that whatever enters fully into the clarity of consciousness is lost for our future inner labours. It can no longer work on the system of our sense organs, on our glandular system or our digestive system, on our nerves, muscles, bones and so on. What enters into consciousness in our soul, what we human beings of today carry within us as the content of our soul, this is something which is no longer at work; it is characterized by the fact that it has become separated from the maternal soil of our total humanity by entering into our consciousness. That which works in the creation of the whole human being is that which exists in the same ratio to these few conscious ideas as do the many fish spawnings in their ratio to the few which become fish.

Whatever is all around us works continually upon our overall human being. Dreams can sometimes teach us how in fact more enters into our soul than what continues to live on in our consciousness, for there are also other impressions which enter the soul. You need only take proper note of the thousands of things which happen in life. In your dream you are in a certain situation. You stand facing a person who is in conversation with someone else; you are the third in the picture. Your dream shows you the face of the person quite clearly, and so on. You say: Where does this dream come from? It seems to be about persons I know in physical life; it is kindled by the physical plane; but where does it come from? I didn't see this or hear that. And then you look into the matter more thoroughly and find that a few days ago you did indeed stand facing that person in a railway carriage, only at the time you were not aware of it. Yet it still lives within you. It is only a lack of accuracy in the way we observe things which causes us not to know something.

The things dreams show us in this way are not particularly important. Other impressions in our soul are much more so. Consider what I told you yesterday about what constantly takes place in human evolution. Human beings have continually been creating Imaginations through their bony system; they have continually been sending Inspirations out into the world through their muscular system, and Intuitions through their nervous system. All this is in the world. Whatever is evil they must atone for through their destiny. But all else fashions and forms the environment of the human being; it continues to be present in our environment. Whatever Imaginations, Inspirations and Intuitions human beings have been sending out into the world since, let's say, the Atlantean catastrophe, all this continues to be present in our environment and is a part of it. It is not necessary for individual human beings to take back into their karma whatever was good in what they have created. What they have sent forth into the spiritual atmosphere of the earth over hundreds and hundreds of centuries in the sequence of epochs continues to live on for present humanity; it is just as present as is the air for physical human beings. Just as we inhale the physical air, just as the air passes from our environment into our physical body, so do the Imaginations, Inspirations and Intuitions pass into us, and we participate in all of them with our soul and spirit.

What is important now is that human beings do not remain unrelated to all they themselves brought forth during earlier epochs of their earthly existence. But they can only become related to all the spiritual content placed by them into the body of the earth if they gradually gain the capacity to absorb these things into their souls.

But how is this done? When we enter into the spiritual meaning of earth's evolution we discover that during the ages in post-Atlantean times when humanity initially still possessed the old clairvoyance, Imaginations, Inspirations and Intuitions continued, generally speaking, to be communicated to the spiritual atmosphere of the earth. That was chiefly the period when those spiritual substances were emitted. Since the fourth post-Atlantean period, but especially from our present time onwards, there will increasingly be less of a sending-out activity and more of a need once again to reabsorb the old with which we are associated and which we originally sent forth. In other words, we are now required to turn an earlier process of spiritual exhalation into one of spiritual inhalation.[31] Human beings must become ever more sensitive to and receptive to the spiritual which is present in the world.

In olden times this was not yet so necessary because it was still possible to put forth spirituality from within; there was still a fund in reserve. But since the fourth post-Atlantean cultural epoch this has been depleted to the extent that in future only what was previously inhaled can, so to speak, be given out again. And it is for this purpose, in order that human beings may knowingly fulfil their new mission within earth existence, that anthroposophy or spiritual science exists. People are drawn to it today not as to some spiritual fad among other fads prevalent nowadays but because it is in its inmost essence bound up with the whole of earthly evolution. That is why humanity must gradually develop an understanding for the spiritual.

Those individuals who from our time onwards fail to develop an understanding of the spirit behind the senses, of the spiritual world which lies behind the sense-perceptible world, will begin to resemble those who have so ruined their respiratory system in their physical body that they can no longer draw breath and therefore suffer from breathlessness. Because a legacy of ancient human wisdom still exists, we are as yet still able to draw on those concepts. But those who in recent times have been observing human evolution with spiritual eyes will see that although material inventions and discoveries are piling up, spiritual content is in the process of becoming completely exhausted. Ever fewer new ideas and new concepts are springing up amongst humanity. Only those who are unfamiliar with the old concepts which they keep on thinking are new discoveries—those who in a way remain immature throughout their lives—can believe that truly new ideas can still arise. The realm of abstract ideas, the realm of intellectual ideas is indeed exhausted. New ideas are no longer springing up.

It was Thales who in a way introduced the earliest intellectual ideas into western thinking.[32] But now we have reached the end; philosophy as the science of ideas is at an end. Human beings must now learn to raise themselves to what lies behind the ideas and thoughts of the physical plane; they must seek what lies beyond this world of ideas. Initially they will raise themselves up to the Imaginations which will once again become a reality for them. This will newly fertilize the spiritual for humanity, and from it, in spiritual science, will flow Imaginations relevant to important universal processes. You need only look at how the description of Saturn, Sun and Moon differs from other things in relation to the abstract concepts of the other sciences. One must give pictorial descriptions of such things so that they cannot be directly realized in the external sense-perceptible world. We describe ancient Saturn as being a state of pure heat. This is nonsense for today's world of sense perceptions; there is no such thing for the sense-perceptible world as a substance consisting of pure heat. But what is nonsense for the world of the senses is true for the world of the spirit; and human beings have the immediate task of entering in a living way into the world of spirit in the very near future.

Those who do not decide to breathe the air of the spirit for which the human soul is to be made receptive through spiritual science—through a science which penetrates beyond what is merely sense-perceptible—

those who do not want to make themselves receptive to the science of the spirit will actually face a state of being which is, in a sense, already coming close to many of us. They will experience a condition of spiritual breathlessness accompanied by spiritual exhaustion which then leads to a spiritual emaciation, a consumptive condition of the spirit.

This would be the fate of those human beings on earth who chose to remain solely in the physical world: to perish through being spiritually consumptive. In the way culture and civilization develop in the future there will be those who are filled with sensitivity, soulfulness and depth of feeling for the spiritual world, for that which initially will be given by spiritual science but which will then arise of its own accord as Imagination, Inspiration and Intuition in human souls. This is what it will be like for one part of humanity; people will have an understanding for and a devotion to the world of spirit. These will be the human beings who fulfil the task with which the earth is now initially confronted.

But others may perhaps remain with the world of the senses; they may not wish to progress beyond the world of the senses or beyond the mere shadow-picture of the sense-perceptible world put forward in philosophical concepts and in external science. These people are moving towards spiritual breathlessness, spiritual emaciation, spiritual infirmity; they will wither within earth existence and not attain the goal set for earth evolution. But earth evolution must allow for every individual to say: Which path shall I choose? In future people will, as it were, tend towards the left or towards the right—those for whom the world of the senses will embrace the whole truth, and those for whom the world of the spirit will encompass the truth.

That the senses, like the human ear, will disappear and that by the end of the earth all earthly senses will have vanished is a fact which can show you how real this emaciation, this withering will be. By relying on the world of the senses we are relying on something which will desert humanity during future earthly evolution. By pressing forward to the world of the spirit we develop ourselves more and more towards what we will encounter during the future of earthly evolution.

A useful symbol for this would be to say: The human being may one day stand there at the end of earthly evolution and speak as does Faust after going blind, for the human being will be not only outwardly blind, but also outwardly deaf, and outwardly without any sense of taste or smell. Yet within him a bright light will shine, and the most wonderful human music and human words will resound.[33] This is what those who have turned towards the spirit will be able to tell. But others, who wanted to remain within the world of the senses, would resemble a Faust who, having lost his sight, would have to say: I am outwardly blind and within me there is no spiritual light; I am entirely enveloped in darkness. Humanity will have to choose between these two Faustian dispositions. The first Faust would have turned towards the world of the spirit, whereas the other Faust would have turned towards the world of the senses and would thus have become familiar with what human beings must feel to be something without essence, something which will have robbed them of their being.

This is what comes into view when we endeavour to bring down from spiritual heights what is immediately necessary for human life. I believe there is no need to describe in words the principles of morality and the impulses of will which, for human beings of the present time, can arise out of a true understanding of spiritual science. Appropriately understood virtue will arise in human hearts out of appropriately comprehended wisdom. If we strive for a true understanding of world evolution, and if we search for wisdom, then the child of wisdom cannot be anything other than love.

It has been the purpose of these lectures to draw your attention to this.

Theosophische Gesellschaft (Adyar)

Deutsche Sektion — Zweig Hannover.

HANNOVER, den 15. November 1911.

Liebe theosophischen Freunde!

Vom 26. Dezember 1911 bis zum 2. Januar 1912 wird Herr Dr. RUDOLF STEINER bei uns anwesend sein, während welcher Zeit die nachfolgenden Veranstaltungen stattfinden:

Am Dienstag, den 26. Dezember 1911 (2. Weihnachtstag) 8 Uhr abends

Weihnachtsfeier,

Vortrag des Herrn Dr. RUDOLF STEINER, in der Aula der neuen höheren Töchterschule I an der Langensalzastrasse.

Von Mittwoch, den 27. Dezember 1911 bis zum Montag, den 1. Januar 1912
8 Uhr abends

Vortrags-Zyklus

des Herrn Dr. RUDOLF STEINER über

„Die Welt der Sinne und die Welt des Geistes"

in der Aula der neuen höheren Töchterschule I an der Langensalzastrasse.

Am Dienstag, den 2. Januar 1912, 8¼ Uhr abends

öffentlicher Vortrag

des Herrn Dr. RUDOLF STEINER über

„Das Wesen der Ewigkeit und die Natur der Menschenseele im Lichte der Geisteswissenschaft"

in der Aula der höheren Schulen am Georgsplatz,

und laden wir hierzu alle Mitglieder der Theosophischen Gesellschaft (Adyar) freundl. ein. In der Hoffnung, recht viele theosophische Mitglieder bei uns begrüssen zu können, zeichnet

mit theosophischem Gruss!

Der Vorstand
des Zweiges Hannover.

Die Teilnehmer an der Weihnachtsfeier und am Zyklus werden gebeten die Karten hierfür, zum Gesamtpreise von M 6.00, bis spätestens zum 5. Dezember d. J. bei Herrn WILH. EGGERS, HANNOVER, Vossstrasse 43, abfordern zu wollen. Karten zum öffentlichen Vortrage sind bei unseren Mitgliedern zu haben. — Wegen Besorgung einer Wohnung wolle man sich gefl. unter Angabe etwaiger Wünsche an Herrn L. ROSENTHAL, HANNOVER, Freytagstrasse 2, wenden.

Theosophical Society (Adyar)

German Section—Hanover Branch

Hanover, 15 November 1911

Dear Theosophical Friends!

From 26 December 1911 to 2 January 1912 Dr RUDOLF STEINER will be present at our meetings, during which time the following events will take place:

On Tuesday, 26 December 1911 (2nd day of Christmas) 8 p.m.

Christmas Festival
Lecture by Dr RUDOLF STEINER in the Assembly Hall of the new Senior Girls' School, I Langensalza Street.

From Wednesday 27 December 1911 to Monday 1 January 1912
8 p.m.

Lecture Cycle
by Dr RUDOLF STEINER on
'The World of the Senses and the World of the Spirit' in the Assembly Hall of the new Senior Girls' School, I Langensalza Street.

On Tuesday 2 January 1912, 8.30 p.m.

Public Lecture
by Dr RUDOLF STEINER on
'The Essence of Eternity and the Nature of the Human Soul
in the Light of Spiritual Science'
in the Assembly Hall of the Senior Schools, Georgen Platz

We warmly invite all members of the
Theosophical Society (Adyar) to attend.
Hoping to greet many theosophical members here, we remain with theosophical greetings

The Executive Council
of the Hanover Branch

Participants at the Christmas Festival and the lecture cycle are requested to obtain tickets (total price 6 Marks) from Herr WILHELM EGGERS, Voss Strasse 43, Hanover latest by 5 December 1911. Tickets for the public lecture may be obtained from our members. Those needing accommodation are advised to contact Herr L. ROSENTHAL, Freytag Strasse 2, Hanover.——

NOTES

Text sources: The lectures in this book were recorded in shorthand by Georg Klenk who also transcribed them into longhand. The original shorthand record is no longer extant. Marie Steiner published the lectures in 1914 in manuscript form and again in 1933 as a book. The third edition was supervised by Dr H.E. Lauer in 1959. The fourth edition (1979) was checked by Caroline Wispler and the fifth (1990) by Susi Lötscher.

As these lectures were given while Rudolf Steiner was still speaking within the auspices of the Theosophical Society, he frequently used the terms 'theosophy' and 'theosophical'. He subsequently indicated that in later editions the terms 'anthroposophy' and 'anthroposophical' should be substituted.

The title: The title of this volume is derived from the title of the lecture series.

The drawings: Rudolf Steiner's drawings on the blackboard were recorded only as they were shown in the original shorthand records. They were redrawn for the 3rd edition by Assja Turgenieff (1890–1966) using the shading technique she had developed.

The German versions of Rudolf Steiner's works mentioned here are shown by their number in the Collected Works (Gesamtausgabe).

1. Rudolf Steiner spoke on this theme in Prague on 19 and 25 March 1911 (published in the journal *Mensch und Welt*, 1968, nos. 1–2 and 3–4) and on 27 and 29 November 1911 in Stuttgart (unpublished). See also the parallel lectures of 31 October and 7 November 1912 in *Ergebnisse der Geistesforschung*, Rudolf Steiner Verlag, Dornach, GA 62.
2. This is a free rendition of a passage in Goethe's *Winckelmann*, chapter 'Antikes', Weimar Edition, Vol. 46, p. 22: 'If the health of a human being is complete, if he feels himself to be a great and comely, a dignified and estimable totality, if his harmonious well-being renders him purely and freely delighted, then the universe, if it were able to have a sense of its own self, would rejoice at having attained its goal and would marvel at the accomplishment of its labours. For what would be served by all that effort of suns and planets and moons, of stars and milky ways, of comets and nebulae, of worlds created and still coming into being, if in the end a joyous human being were not unconsciously to delight in his own existence?'
3. Chorus from *Antigone* by Sophocles, Verses 332.
4. See for example the 'Supplement' to a letter from Goethe to Zelter dated 22 June 1808: '... In this way the human being is so exalted that what otherwise cannot be depicted is, in fact, depicted in him. What is the string of an

instrument or any mechanical division thereof in comparison with the musician's ear? ...' (Also included in the chapter 'Sayings in Prose' in Goethe's *Scientific Writings* edited and annotated by Rudolf Steiner in Kürschner's *Deutsche National-Litteratur*, 5 volumes, 1884–97, reprinted Dornach 1975 (GA 1a–e, Vol. 5, p. 351), and in Goethe, *Maximen und Reflexionen*, Maxim 708.

5. Laurenz Müllner (b. July 1848 at Gross-Grillowitz, d. 28 November 1911 at Merano). In the monthly journal *Anthroposophie. Monatsschrift für freies Geistesleben* (1933, Book 1), C.S. Picht was able to quote from an obituary (manuscript) written by the poet Marie Eugenie delle Grazie who had been Müllner's friend: 'Cardinals Rauscher and Kutschker, and also the distinguished church historian Karl Werner, were very favourably disposed towards Müllner's efforts. Consequently, on 29 September 1880, the Ministry for Cultural Affairs and Education commissioned him to lecture on theological philosophy at Vienna University's theological faculty. In 1883 he was appointed professor extraordinary of Christian philosophy. Müllner spent the winter of 1886/87 in Rome where he was obliged to defend himself against a denunciation of his "anti-ecclesiastical philosophy". Pope Leo XIII, more open-minded and far-sighted than Müllner's opponents, advised "the German idealist" to pay a visit to certain Thomistic colleagues and "in addition to have a good look about him Rome"! Thus exonerated of suspected latent heretical tendencies, Müllner returned to Vienna where he was then appointed professor in ordinary of Christian philosophy.' See also Rudolf Steiner on Laurenz Müllner in *The Course of My Life*, Chapter VII, Anthroposophic Press, New York 1990 (GA 28) and in *The Riddle of Man; From the Thinking, Observations, and Contemplations of a Series of German and Austrian Personalities*, Mercury Press, New York 1990 (GA 20).
6. See Plato, the *Theaetetus*, 155 D: '... for this is the state of mind of a man (a philosopher) greatly devoted to wisdom: to be amazed. For there is no other inauguration for the love of wisdom (philosophy) than this.' See also Aristotle, the *Metaphysics*, 982b, First Book (A), Chapter 2: 'When human beings now, and in the past, began to think philosophically, what gave them the impetus for this was amazement, initially about matters close at hand, and then about those further in the past, so that they also pondered upon the phases of the moon, or the course of the sun and the stars, and also upon the origins of the universe.'
7. In general, Rudolf Steiner refers to these as the seven members of the human being: physical body, ether body, astral body, 'I', Spirit Self, Life Spirit, Spirit Man.
8. This reference is to Valentinus, the Gnostic teacher who founded the Valentinian sect. There is a chapter on Valentinus in the book *Die Gnosis. Grundlagen der Weltanschauung einer edleren Kultur* (Leipzig 1903) by Eugen Heinrich Schmitt, a friend of Rudolf Steiner.
9. 'First and foremost one must understand that everything factual is theoretical... One should not look for what is behind the phenomena; they themselves are the instruction.' See 'Sayings in Prose' in Goethe's *Scientific Writings* edited and annotated by Rudolf Steiner in Kürschner's *Deutsche*

National-Litteratur, 5 volumes, 1884–97, reprinted Dornach 1975 (in GA 1a–e, Vol. 5, p. 376). Rudolf Steiner wrote about this in his 'Introduction' to the 'Sayings in Prose', ibid. pp. 339ff. (Also in Rudolf Steiner *Einleitungen zu Goethes Naturwissenschaftlichen Schriften* (1884–97) (in GA 1, Chapter XVIII and in Goethe *Maximen und Reflexionen*, Maxim 575.)

10. Immanuel Kant in *Critique of Pure Reason*, Part II, Section II, Book II, Transcendental Dialectic (translation by J.M.D. Meiklejohn): 'If, then, I could understand the nature of a cosmological idea, and perceive, before I entered on the discussion of the subject at all, that, whatever side of the question regarding the unconditioned of the regressive synthesis of phenomena it favoured, it must either be *too great* or *too small* for every *conception of the understanding*; I would be able to comprehend how the idea, which relates to an object of experience—an experience which must be adequate to and in accordance with a possible conception of the understanding—must be completely void and without significance, inasmuch as its object is inadequate, consider it as we may. And this is actually the case with all cosmological conceptions which, for the reason above-mentioned, involve reason, so long as it remains attached to them, in an unavoidable antinomy. For suppose: *first*, that *the world has no beginning*—in this case it is *too large* for our conception; for this conception, which consists in a successive Regressus, cannot overtake the whole eternity that has elapsed. Grant that *it has a beginning*, it is then *too small* for the conception of the understanding. For, as a beginning presupposed a time preceding, it cannot be unconditioned; and the law of the empirical employment of the understanding imposes the necessity of looking for a higher condition of time; and the world is, therefore, evidently *too small* for this law.' See also op. cit.: Antinomy of Pure Reason, Chapter 7, 'Sceptical Exposition of the Cosmological Problems'.
11. See Vincenz Knauer, *Die Hauptprobleme der Philosophie in ihrer Entwicklung und teilweisen Lösung von Thales bis Robert Hamerling*, lectures given at the University of Vienna, Vienna & Leipzig 1892, pp. 136f, 21st lecture, 1. 'The Sources of Knowledge': '... The wolf, for example, consists of physical components identical to those of the lamb; its physical body is built from the assimilated flesh of the lamb; yet the wolf does not become a lamb even if it spends its whole life eating nothing but lambs. So what makes it a wolf must of course be something other than sense-perceptible matter; it must not and cannot be merely an idea in the mind even though it is only accessible through thinking and not through the senses; it must be a reality, something real.'
12. Arthur Schopenhauer, 1788–1860, philosopher, *The World as Will and Idea*, Book 3, paragraph 52; *Schopenhauers sämtliche Werke*, edited and with an introduction by Rudolf Steiner, Stuttgart, no date, Volume 3, pp. 105ff: '... Music is as *direct* an objectivation and image of the whole *will* as is the world itself, indeed as are the ideas of which the many and varied manifestations portray the separate things of the world. So music is in no way, as are the other arts, an image of the ideas; it is an *image of the will* of which the ideas are also the objectivity. That is why the effect of music is so very much more powerful and penetrating than that of the other arts, which speak only of the shadow, whereas music speaks of the inherent being ...'

13. See 'The Metamorphosis of Plants' in Goethe's *Scientific Writings* edited and annotated by Rudolf Steiner in Kürschner's *Deutsche National-Litteratur*, 5 volumes, 1884–97, reprinted Dornach 1975 (GA 1a–e, Vol. 1, pp. 17ff, and Rudolf Steiner's 'Introduction' in the same volume.
14. See more in Lecture Six in the present volume. Rudolf Steiner also spoke about this in, among others, *Rosicrucian Wisdom*, Rudolf Steiner Press, London 2000, 14 lectures, Munich 1907 (GA 99), lecture of 5 June; and in *Menschheitsentwicklung und Christus-Erkenntnis*, Rudolf Steiner Verlag, Dornach, 22 lectures, Kassel and Basel 1907 (GA 100), lectures of 28 and 29 June.
15. Rudolf Steiner, *How to Know Higher Worlds*, Anthroposopohic Press, New York 1994 (GA 10).
16. Genesis, 3,5.
17. Regarding the development of the 12 senses see also Rudolf Steiner's description in *The Riddle of Humanity, The Spiritual Background of Human History*, Rudolf Steiner Press, London 1990 (GA 170), Lecture 14.
18. See Note 15.
19. Dr Carl Unger, 1878–1929, member of the Executive Council of the Anthroposophical Society, and a pupil of Rudolf Steiner. See especially 'Die Grundlehren der Anthroposophie' (1910–11) in *Schriften*, Vol. 1, Stuttgart 1964.
20. Rudolf Steiner, *The Philosophy of Freedom*, Rudolf Steiner Press, London 1970 (GA 4).
21. See Rudolf Steiner, *From Jesus to Christ*, Rudolf Steiner Press, London 1973 (GA 131).
22. See Rudolf Steiner *An Outline of Esoteric Science*, (1910), Rudolf Steiner Press, London 1969 (GA 13), Chapter 'Man and the Evolution of the World'.
23. See Note 15.
24. In Goethe's *Faust, Part I*, The Study, line 1740, it is Mephistopheles who utters the sentence: 'Blood is a juice of rarest quality!' See also Rudolf Steiner's lecture of 25 October 1906, *The Occult Significance of Blood*, Rudolf Steiner Press, London 1967 (in GA 55).
25. *Faust, Part I*, The Study, lines 1737–40.
26. Rudolf Steiner, *Genesis, Secrets of Creation*, Munich 1910, Rudolf Steiner Press, Forest Row 2000 (GA 122).
27. Regarding the healing powers of metals see Rudolf Steiner, *True and False Paths in Spiritual Investigation*, Torquay 1924, Rudolf Steiner Press, London 1969 (GA 243).
28. See, for example, B. Gustav Theodor Fechner, *Nanna oder über das Seelenleben der Pflanzen*, Leipzig 1848; or Raoul Francé, *Das Sinnesleben der Pflanzen*, Stuttgart 1905.
29. See Goethe's *Faust, Part II*, Act 1, A Gloomy Gallery, lines 6211 ff.
30. Charles Darwin (1809–82), English naturalist, physician, botanist and geologist. His main work: *On the Origin of Species by Means of Natural Selection, or the Preservation of Favoured Races in the Struggle for Life*, London 1859.
31. See also Rudolf Steiner's lecture of 13 January 1924 in *Rosicrucianism and Modern Initiation*, Rudolf Steiner Press, London 1965 (in GA 233a).

32. Thales (*c.* 625–545 BC). See also Rudolf Steiner, *The Riddles of Philosophy*, Anthroposophic Press, New York 1973 (GA 18).
33. See Goethe's *Faust, Part II*, Act 5, Midnight, line 11500.

RUDOLF STEINER'S COLLECTED WORKS

The German Edition of Rudolf Steiner's Collected Works (the *Gesamtausgabe* [GA] published by Rudolf Steiner Verlag, Dornach, Switzerland) presently runs to 354 titles, organized either by type of work (written or spoken), chronology, audience (public or other), or subject (education, art, etc.). For ease of comparison, the Collected Works in English [CW] follows the German organization exactly. A complete listing of the CWs follows with literal translations of the German titles. Other than in the case of the books published in his lifetime, titles were rarely given by Rudolf Steiner himself, and were often provided by the editors of the German editions. The titles in English are not necessarily the same as the German; and, indeed, over the past seventy-five years have frequently been different, with the same book sometimes appearing under different titles.

For ease of identification and to avoid confusion, we suggest that readers looking for a title should do so by CW number. Because the work of creating the Collected Works of Rudolf Steiner is an ongoing process, with new titles being published every year, we have not indicated in this listing which books are presently available. To find out what titles in the Collected Works are currently in print, please check our website at www.rudolfsteinerpress.com (or www.steinerbooks.org for US readers).

Written Work

CW 1	Goethe: Natural-Scientific Writings, Introduction, with Footnotes and Explanations in the text by Rudolf Steiner
CW 2	Outlines of an Epistemology of the Goethean World View, with Special Consideration of Schiller
CW 3	Truth and Science
CW 4	The Philosophy of Freedom
CW 4a	Documents to 'The Philosophy of Freedom'
CW 5	Friedrich Nietzsche, A Fighter against His Own Time
CW 6	Goethe's Worldview
CW 6a	Now in CW 30
CW 7	Mysticism at the Dawn of Modern Spiritual Life and Its Relationship with Modern Worldviews
CW 8	Christianity as Mystical Fact and the Mysteries of Antiquity
CW 9	Theosophy: An Introduction into Supersensible World Knowledge and Human Purpose
CW 10	How Does One Attain Knowledge of Higher Worlds?
CW 11	From the Akasha-Chronicle

CW 12	Levels of Higher Knowledge
CW 13	Occult Science in Outline
CW 14	Four Mystery Dramas
CW 15	The Spiritual Guidance of the Individual and Humanity
CW 16	A Way to Human Self-Knowledge: Eight Meditations
CW 17	The Threshold of the Spiritual World. Aphoristic Comments
CW 18	The Riddles of Philosophy in Their History, Presented as an Outline
CW 19	Contained in CW 24
CW 20	The Riddles of the Human Being: Articulated and Unarticulated in the Thinking, Views and Opinions of a Series of German and Austrian Personalities
CW 21	The Riddles of the Soul
CW 22	Goethe's Spiritual Nature And Its Revelation In 'Faust' and through the 'Fairy Tale of the Snake and the Lily'
CW 23	The Central Points of the Social Question in the Necessities of Life in the Present and the Future
CW 24	Essays Concerning the Threefold Division of the Social Organism and the Period 1915–1921
CW 25	Cosmology, Religion and Philosophy
CW 26	Anthroposophical Leading Thoughts
CW 27	Fundamentals for Expansion of the Art of Healing according to Spiritual-Scientific Insights
CW 28	The Course of My Life
CW 29	Collected Essays on Dramaturgy, 1889–1900
CW 30	Methodical Foundations of Anthroposophy: Collected Essays on Philosophy, Natural Science, Aesthetics and Psychology, 1884–1901
CW 31	Collected Essays on Culture and Current Events, 1887–1901
CW 32	Collected Essays on Literature, 1884–1902
CW 33	Biographies and Biographical Sketches, 1894–1905
CW 34	Lucifer-Gnosis: Foundational Essays on Anthroposophy and Reports from the Periodicals 'Lucifer' and 'Lucifer-Gnosis,' 1903–1908
CW 35	Philosophy and Anthroposophy: Collected Essays, 1904–1923
CW 36	The Goetheanum-Idea in the Middle of the Cultural Crisis of the Present: Collected Essays from the Periodical 'Das Goetheanum,' 1921–1925
CW 37	Now in CWs 260a and 251
CW 38	Letters, Vol. 1: 1881–1890
CW 39	Letters, Vol. 2: 1890–1925
CW 40	Truth-Wrought Words
CW 40a	Sayings, Poems and Mantras; Supplementary Volume
CW 42	Now in CWs 264–266
CW 43	Stage Adaptations
CW 44	On the Four Mystery Dramas. Sketches, Fragments and Paralipomena on the Four Mystery Dramas
CW 45	Anthroposophy: A Fragment from the Year 1910

Public Lectures

CW 51	On Philosophy, History and Literature
CW 52	Spiritual Teachings Concerning the Soul and Observation of the World
CW 53	The Origin and Goal of the Human Being
CW 54	The Riddles of the World and Anthroposophy
CW 55	Knowledge of the Supersensible in Our Times and Its Meaning for Life Today
CW 56	Knowledge of the Soul and of the Spirit
CW 57	Where and How Does One Find the Spirit?
CW 58	The Metamorphoses of the Soul Life. Paths of Soul Experiences: Part One
CW 59	The Metamorphoses of the Soul Life. Paths of Soul Experiences: Part Two
CW 60	The Answers of Spiritual Science to the Biggest Questions of Existence
CW 61	Human History in the Light of Spiritual Research
CW 62	Results of Spiritual Research
CW 63	Spiritual Science as a Treasure for Life
CW 64	Out of Destiny-Burdened Times
CW 65	Out of Central European Spiritual Life
CW 66	Spirit and Matter, Life and Death
CW 67	The Eternal in the Human Soul. Immortality and Freedom
CW 68	Public lectures in various cities, 1906–1918
CW 69	Public lectures in various cities, 1906–1918
CW 70	Public lectures in various cities, 1906–1918
CW 71	Public lectures in various cities, 1906–1918
CW 72	Freedom—Immortality—Social Life
CW 73	The Supplementing of the Modern Sciences through Anthroposophy
CW 73a	Specialized Fields of Knowledge and Anthroposophy
CW 74	The Philosophy of Thomas Aquinas
CW 75	Public lectures in various cities, 1906–1918
CW 76	The Fructifying Effect of Anthroposophy on Specialized Fields
CW 77a	The Task of Anthroposophy in Relation to Science and Life: The Darmstadt College Course
CW 77b	Art and Anthroposophy. The Goetheanum-Impulse
CW 78	Anthroposophy, Its Roots of Knowledge and Fruits for Life
CW 79	The Reality of the Higher Worlds
CW 80	Public lectures in various cities, 1922
CW 81	Renewal-Impulses for Culture and Science—Berlin College Course
CW 82	So that the Human Being Can Become a Complete Human Being
CW 83	Western and Eastern World-Contrast. Paths to Understanding It through Anthroposophy
CW 84	What Did the Goetheanum Intend and What Should Anthroposophy Do?

Lectures to the Members of the Anthroposophical Society

CW 88	Concerning the Astral World and Devachan
CW 89	Consciousness—Life—Form. Fundamental Principles of a Spiritual-Scientific Cosmology
CW 90	Participant Notes from the Lectures during the Years 1903–1905
CW 91	Participant Notes from the Lectures during the Years 1903–1905
CW 92	The Occult Truths of Ancient Myths and Sagas
CW 93	The Temple Legend and the Golden Legend
CW 93a	Fundamentals of Esotericism
CW 94	Cosmogony. Popular Occultism. The Gospel of John. The Theosophy in the Gospel of John
CW 95	At the Gates of Theosophy
CW 96	Origin-Impulses of Spiritual Science. Christian Esotericism in the Light of New Spirit-Knowledge
CW 97	The Christian Mystery
CW 98	Nature Beings and Spirit Beings—Their Effects in Our Visible World
CW 99	The Theosophy of the Rosicrucians
CW 100	Human Development and Christ-Knowledge
CW 101	Myths and Legends. Occult Signs and Symbols
CW 102	The Working into Human Beings by Spiritual Beings
CW 103	The Gospel of John
CW 104	The Apocalypse of John
CW 104a	From the Picture-Script of the Apocalypse of John
CW 105	Universe, Earth, the Human Being: Their Being and Development, as well as Their Reflection in the Connection between Egyptian Mythology and Modern Culture
CW 106	Egyptian Myths and Mysteries in Relation to the Active Spiritual Forces of the Present
CW 107	Spiritual-Scientific Knowledge of the Human Being
CW 108	Answering the Questions of Life and the World through Anthroposophy
CW 109	The Principle of Spiritual Economy in Connection with the Question of Reincarnation. An Aspect of the Spiritual Guidance of Humanity
CW 110	The Spiritual Hierarchies and Their Reflection in the Physical World. Zodiac, Planets and Cosmos
CW 111	Contained in CW 109
CW 112	The Gospel of John in Relation to the Three Other Gospels, Especially the Gospel of Luke
CW 113	The Orient in the Light of the Occident. The Children of Lucifer and the Brothers of Christ
CW 114	The Gospel of Luke
CW 115	Anthroposophy—Psychosophy—Pneumatosophy
CW 116	The Christ-Impulse and the Development of 'I'-Consciousness
CW 117	The Deeper Secrets of the Development of Humanity in Light of the Gospels

CW 118 The Event of the Christ-Appearance in the Etheric World
CW 119 Macrocosm and Microcosm. The Large World and the Small World. Soul-Questions, Life-Questions, Spirit-Questions
CW 120 The Revelation of Karma
CW 121 The Mission of Individual Folk-Souls in Connection with Germanic-Nordic Mythology
CW 122 The Secrets of the Biblical Creation-Story. The Six-Day Work in the First Book of Moses
CW 123 The Gospel of Matthew
CW 124 Excursus in the Area of the Gospel of Mark
CW 125 Paths and Goals of the Spiritual Human Being. Life Questions in the Light of Spiritual Science
CW 126 Occult History. Esoteric Observations of the Karmic Relationships of Personalities and Events of World History
CW 127 The Mission of the New Spiritual Revelation. The Christ-Event as the Middle-Point of Earth Evolution
CW 128 An Occult Physiology
CW 129 Wonders of the World, Trials of the Soul, and Revelations of the Spirit
CW 130 Esoteric Christianity and the Spiritual Guidance of Humanity
CW 131 From Jesus to Christ
CW 132 Evolution from the View Point of the Truth
CW 133 The Earthly and the Cosmic Human Being
CW 134 The World of the Senses and the World of the Spirit
CW 135 Reincarnation and Karma and their Meaning for the Culture of the Present
CW 136 The Spiritual Beings in Celestial Bodies and the Realms of Nature
CW 137 The Human Being in the Light of Occultism, Theosophy and Philosophy
CW 138 On Initiation. On Eternity and the Passing Moment. On the Light of the Spirit and the Darkness of Life
CW 139 The Gospel of Mark
CW 140 Occult Investigation into the Life between Death and New Birth. The Living Interaction between Life and Death
CW 141 Life between Death and New Birth in Relationship to Cosmic Facts
CW 142 The Bhagavad Gita and the Letters of Paul
CW 143 Experiences of the Supersensible. Three Paths of the Soul to Christ
CW 144 The Mysteries of the East and of Christianity
CW 145 What Significance Does Occult Development of the Human Being Have for the Sheaths—Physical Body, Etheric Body, Astral Body, and Self?
CW 146 The Occult Foundations of the Bhagavad Gita
CW 147 The Secrets of the Threshold
CW 148 Out of Research in the Akasha: The Fifth Gospel
CW 149 Christ and the Spiritual World. Concerning the Search for the Holy Grail

CW 150	The World of the Spirit and Its Extension into Physical Existence; The Influence of the Dead in the World of the Living
CW 151	Human Thought and Cosmic Thought
CW 152	Preliminary Stages to the Mystery of Golgotha
CW 153	The Inner Being of the Human Being and Life Between Death and New Birth
CW 154	How does One Gain an Understanding of the Spiritual World? The Flowing in of Spiritual Impulses from out of the World of the Deceased
CW 155	Christ and the Human Soul. Concerning the Meaning of Life. Theosophical Morality. Anthroposophy and Christianity
CW 156	Occult Reading and Occult Hearing
CW 157	Human Destinies and the Destiny of Peoples
CW 157a	The Formation of Destiny and the Life after Death
CW 158	The Connection Between the Human Being and the Elemental World. Kalevala—Olaf Åsteson—The Russian People—The World as the Result of the Influences of Equilibrium
CW 159	The Mystery of Death. The Nature and Significance of Middle Europe and the European Folk Spirits
CW 160	In CW 159
CW 161	Paths of Spiritual Knowledge and the Renewal of the Artistic Worldview
CW 162	Questions of Art and Life in Light of Spiritual Science
CW 163	Coincidence, Necessity and Providence. Imaginative Knowledge and the Processes after Death
CW 164	The Value of Thinking for a Knowledge That Satisfies the Human Being. The Relationship of Spiritual Science to Natural Science
CW 165	The Spiritual Unification of Humanity through the Christ-Impulse
CW 166	Necessity and Freedom in the Events of the World and in Human Action
CW 167	The Present and the Past in the Human Spirit
CW 168	The Connection between the Living and the Dead
CW 169	World-being and Selfhood
CW 170	The Riddle of the Human Being. The Spiritual Background of Human History. Cosmic and Human History, Vol. 1
CW 171	Inner Development-Impulses of Humanity. Goethe and the Crisis of the 19th Century. Cosmic and Human History, Vol. 2
CW 172	The Karma of the Vocation of the Human Being in Connection with Goethe's Life. Cosmic and Human History, Vol. 3
CW 173	Contemporary-Historical Considerations: The Karma of Untruthfulness, Part One. Cosmic and Human History, Vol. 4
CW 174	Contemporary-Historical Considerations: The Karma of Untruthfulness, Part Two. Cosmic and Human History, Vol. 5
CW 174a	Middle Europe between East and West. Cosmic and Human History, Vol. 6
CW 174b	The Spiritual Background of the First World War. Cosmic and Human History, Vol. 7

CW 175	Building Stones for an Understanding of the Mystery of Golgotha. Cosmic and Human Metamorphoses
CW 176	Truths of Evolution of the Individual and Humanity. The Karma of Materialism
CW 177	The Spiritual Background of the Outer World. The Fall of the Spirits of Darkness. Spiritual Beings and Their Effects, Vol. 1
CW 178	Individual Spiritual Beings and their Influence in the Soul of the Human Being. Spiritual Beings and their Effects, Vol. 2
CW 179	Spiritual Beings and Their Effects. Historical Necessity and Freedom. The Influences on Destiny from out of the World of the Dead. Spiritual Beings and Their Effects, Vol. 3
CW 180	Mystery Truths and Christmas Impulses. Ancient Myths and their Meaning. Spiritual Beings and Their Effects, Vol. 4
CW 181	Earthly Death and Cosmic Life. Anthroposophical Gifts for Life. Necessities of Consciousness for the Present and the Future.
CW 182	Death as Transformation of Life
CW 183	The Science of the Development of the Human Being
CW 184	The Polarity of Duration and Development in Human Life. The Cosmic Pre-History of Humanity
CW 185	Historical Symptomology
CW 185a	Historical-Developmental Foundations for Forming a Social Judgement
CW 186	The Fundamental Social Demands of Our Time—In Changed Situations
CW 187	How Can Humanity Find the Christ Again? The Threefold Shadow-Existence of our Time and the New Christ-Light
CW 188	Goetheanism, a Transformation-Impulse and Resurrection-Thought. Science of the Human Being and Science of Sociology
CW 189	The Social Question as a Question of Consciousness. The Spiritual Background of the Social Question, Vol. 1
CW 190	Impulses of the Past and the Future in Social Occurrences. The Spiritual Background of the Social Question, Vol. 2
CW 191	Social Understanding from Spiritual-Scientific Cognition. The Spiritual Background of the Social Question, Vol. 3
CW 192	Spiritual-Scientific Treatment of Social and Pedagogical Questions
CW 193	The Inner Aspect of the Social Riddle. Luciferic Past and Ahrimanic Future
CW 194	The Mission of Michael. The Revelation of the Actual Mysteries of the Human Being
CW 195	Cosmic New Year and the New Year Idea
CW 196	Spiritual and Social Transformations in the Development of Humanity
CW 197	Polarities in the Development of Humanity: West and East Materialism and Mysticism Knowledge and Belief
CW 198	Healing Factors for the Social Organism
CW 199	Spiritual Science as Knowledge of the Foundational Impulses of Social Formation

CW 200	The New Spirituality and the Christ-Experience of the 20th Century
CW 201	The Correspondences Between Microcosm and Macrocosm. The Human Being—A Hieroglyph of the Universe. The Human Being in Relationship with the Cosmos: 1
CW 202	The Bridge between the World-Spirituality and the Physical Aspect of the Human Being. The Search for the New Isis, the Divine Sophia. The Human Being in Relationship with the Cosmos: 2
CW 203	The Responsibility of Human Beings for the Development of the World through their Spiritual Connection with the Planet Earth and the World of the Stars. The Human Being in Relationship with the Cosmos: 3
CW 204	Perspectives of the Development of Humanity. The Materialistic Knowledge-Impulse and the Task of Anthroposophy. The Human Being in Relationship with the Cosmos: 4
CW 205	Human Development, World-Soul, and World-Spirit. Part One: The Human Being as a Being of Body and Soul in Relationship to the World. The Human Being in Relationship with the Cosmos: 5
CW 206	Human Development, World-Soul, and World-Spirit. Part Two: The Human Being as a Spiritual Being in the Process of Historical Development. The Human Being in Relationship with the Cosmos: 6
CW 207	Anthroposophy as Cosmosophy. Part One: Characteristic Features of the Human Being in the Earthly and the Cosmic Realms. The Human Being in Relationship with the Cosmos: 7
CW 208	Anthroposophy as Cosmosophy. Part Two: The Forming of the Human Being as the Result of Cosmic Influence. The Human Being in Relationship with the Cosmos: 8
CW 209	Nordic and Central European Spiritual Impulses. The Festival of the Appearance of Christ. The Human Being in Relationship with the Cosmos: 9
CW 210	Old and New Methods of Initiation. Drama and Poetry in the Change of Consciousness in the Modern Age
CW 211	The Sun Mystery and the Mystery of Death and Resurrection. Exoteric and Esoteric Christianity
CW 212	Human Soul Life and Spiritual Striving in Connection with World and Earth Development
CW 213	Human Questions and World Answers
CW 214	The Mystery of the Trinity: The Human Being in Relationship with the Spiritual World in the Course of Time
CW 215	Philosophy, Cosmology, and Religion in Anthroposophy
CW 216	The Fundamental Impulses of the World-Historical Development of Humanity
CW 217	Spiritually Active Forces in the Coexistence of the Older and Younger Generations. Pedagogical Course for Youth

CW 217a	Youth's Cognitive Task
CW 218	Spiritual Connections in the Forming of the Human Organism
CW 219	The Relationship of the World of the Stars to the Human Being, and of the Human Being to the World of the Stars. The Spiritual Communion of Humanity
CW 220	Living Knowledge of Nature. Intellectual Fall and Spiritual Redemption
CW 221	Earth-Knowing and Heaven-Insight
CW 222	The Imparting of Impulses to World-Historical Events through Spiritual Powers
CW 223	The Cycle of the Year as Breathing Process of the Earth and the Four Great Festival-Seasons. Anthroposophy and the Human Heart (Gemüt)
CW 224	The Human Soul and its Connection with Divine-Spiritual Individualities. The Internalization of the Festivals of the Year
CW 225	Three Perspectives of Anthroposophy. Cultural Phenomena observed from a Spiritual-Scientific Perspective
CW 226	Human Being, Human Destiny, and World Development
CW 227	Initiation-Knowledge
CW 228	Science of Initiation and Knowledge of the Stars. The Human Being in the Past, the Present, and the Future from the Viewpoint of the Development of Consciousness
CW 229	The Experiencing of the Course of the Year in Four Cosmic Imaginations
CW 230	The Human Being as Harmony of the Creative, Building, and Formative World-Word
CW 231	The Supersensible Human Being, Understood Anthroposophically
CW 232	The Forming of the Mysteries
CW 233	World History Illuminated by Anthroposophy and as the Foundation for Knowledge of the Human Spirit
CW 233a	Mystery Sites of the Middle Ages: Rosicrucianism and the Modern Initiation-Principle. The Festival of Easter as Part of the History of the Mysteries of Humanity
CW 234	Anthroposophy. A Summary after 21 Years
CW 235	Esoteric Observations of Karmic Relationships in 6 Volumes, Vol. 1
CW 236	Esoteric Observations of Karmic Relationships in 6 Volumes, Vol. 2
CW 237	Esoteric Observations of Karmic Relationships in 6 Volumes, Vol. 3: The Karmic Relationships of the Anthroposophical Movement
CW 238	Esoteric Observations of Karmic Relationships in 6 Volumes, Vol. 4: The Spiritual Life of the Present in Relationship to the Anthroposophical Movement
CW 239	Esoteric Observations of Karmic Relationships in 6 Volumes, Vol. 5

CW 240	Esoteric Observations of Karmic Relationships in 6 Volumes, Vol. 6
CW 243	The Consciousness of the Initiate
CW 245	Instructions for an Esoteric Schooling
CW 250	The Building-Up of the Anthroposophical Society. From the Beginning to the Outbreak of the First World War
CW 251	The History of the Goetheanum Building-Association
CW 252	Life in the Anthroposophical Society from the First World War to the Burning of the First Goetheanum
CW 253	The Problems of Living Together in the Anthroposophical Society. On the Dornach Crisis of 1915. With Highlights on Swedenborg's Clairvoyance, the Views of Freudian Psychoanalysts, and the Concept of Love in Relation to Mysticism
CW 254	The Occult Movement in the 19th Century and Its Relationship to World Culture. Significant Points from the Exoteric Cultural Life around the Middle of the 19th Century
CW 255	Rudolf Steiner during the First World War
CW 255a	Anthroposophy and the Reformation of Society. On the History of the Threefold Movement
CW 255b	Anthroposophy and Its Opponents, 1919–1921
CW 256	How Can the Anthroposophical Movement Be Financed?
CW 256a	Futurum, Inc. / International Laboratories, Inc.
CW 256b	The Coming Day, Inc.
CW 257	Anthroposophical Community-Building
CW 258	The History of and Conditions for the Anthroposophical Movement in Relationship to the Anthroposophical Society. A Stimulus to Self-Contemplation
CW 259	The Year of Destiny 1923 in the History of the Anthroposophical Society. From the Burning of the Goetheanum to the Christmas Conference
CW 260	The Christmas Conference for the Founding of the General Anthroposophical Society
CW 260a	The Constitution of the General Anthroposophical Society and the School for Spiritual Science. The Rebuilding of the Goetheanum
CW 261	Our Dead. Addresses, Words of Remembrance, and Meditative Verses, 1906–1924
CW 262	Rudolf Steiner and Marie Steiner-von Sivers: Correspondence and Documents, 1901–1925
CW 263/1	Rudolf Steiner and Edith Maryon: Correspondence: Letters, Verses, Sketches, 1912–1924
CW 264	On the History and the Contents of the First Section of the Esoteric School from 1904 to 1914. Letters, Newsletters, Documents, Lectures
CW 265	On the History and from the Contents of the Ritual-Knowledge Section of the Esoteric School from 1904 to 1914. Documents, and Lectures from the Years 1906 to 1914, as Well as on New Approaches to Ritual-Knowledge Work in the Years 1921–1924

CW 266/1	From the Contents of the Esoteric Lessons. Volume 1: 1904–1909. Notes from Memory of Participants. Meditation texts from the notes of Rudolf Steiner
CW 266/2	From the Contents of the Esoteric Lessons. Volume 2: 1910–1912. Notes from Memory of Participants
CW 266/3	From the Contents of the Esoteric Lessons. Volume 3: 1913, 1914 and 1920–1923. Notes from Memory of Participants. Meditation texts from the notes of Rudolf Steiner
CW 267	Soul-Exercises: Vol. 1: Exercises with Word and Image Meditations for the Methodological Development of Higher Powers of Knowledge, 1904–1924
CW 268	Soul-Exercises: Vol. 2: Mantric Verses, 1903–1925
CW 269	Ritual Texts for the Celebration of the Free Christian Religious Instruction. The Collected Verses for Teachers and Students of the Waldorf School
CW 270	Esoteric Instructions for the First Class of the School for Spiritual Science at the Goetheanum 1924, 4 Volumes
CW 271	Art and Knowledge of Art. Foundations of a New Aesthetic
CW 272	Spiritual-Scientific Commentary on Goethe's 'Faust' in Two Volumes. Vol. 1: Faust, the Striving Human Being
CW 273	Spiritual-Scientific Commentary on Goethe's 'Faust' in Two Volumes. Vol. 2: The Faust-Problem
CW 274	Addresses for the Christmas Plays from the Old Folk Traditions
CW 275	Art in the Light of Mystery-Wisdom
CW 276	The Artistic in Its Mission in the World. The Genius of Language. The World of Self-Revealing Radiant Appearances—Anthroposophy and Art. Anthroposophy and Poetry
CW 277	Eurythmy. The Revelation of the Speaking Soul
CW 277a	The Origin and Development of Eurythmy
CW 278	Eurythmy as Visible Song
CW 279	Eurythmy as Visible Speech
CW 280	The Method and Nature of Speech Formation
CW 281	The Art of Recitation and Declamation
CW 282	Speech Formation and Dramatic Art
CW 283	The Nature of Things Musical and the Experience of Tone in the Human Being
CW 284/285	Images of Occult Seals and Pillars. The Munich Congress of Whitsun 1907 and Its Consequences
CW 286	Paths to a New Style of Architecture. 'And the Building Becomes Human'
CW 287	The Building at Dornach as a Symbol of Historical Becoming and an Artistic Transformation Impulse
CW 288	Style-Forms in the Living Organic
CW 289	The Building-Idea of the Goetheanum: Lectures with Slides from the Years 1920–1921
CW 290	The Building-Idea of the Goetheanum: Lectures with Slides from the Years 1920–1921

CW 291	The Nature of Colours
CW 291a	Knowledge of Colours. Supplementary Volume to 'The Nature of Colours'
CW 292	Art History as Image of Inner Spiritual Impulses
CW 293	General Knowledge of the Human Being as the Foundation of Pedagogy
CW 294	The Art of Education, Methodology and Didactics
CW 295	The Art of Education: Seminar Discussions and Lectures on Lesson Planning
CW 296	The Question of Education as a Social Question
CW 297	The Idea and Practice of the Waldorf School
CW 297a	Education for Life: Self-Education and the Practice of Pedagogy
CW 298	Rudolf Steiner in the Waldorf School
CW 299	Spiritual-Scientific Observations on Speech
CW 300a	Conferences with the Teachers of the Free Waldorf School in Stuttgart, 1919 to 1924, in 3 Volumes, Vol. 1
CW 300b	Conferences with the Teachers of the Free Waldorf School in Stuttgart, 1919 to 1924, in 3 Volumes, Vol. 2
CW 300c	Conferences with the Teachers of the Free Waldorf School in Stuttgart, 1919 to 1924, in 3 Volumes, Vol. 3
CW 301	The Renewal of Pedagogical-Didactical Art through Spiritual Science
CW 302	Knowledge of the Human Being and the Forming of Class Lessons
CW 302a	Education and Teaching from a Knowledge of the Human Being
CW 303	The Healthy Development of the Human Being
CW 304	Methods of Education and Teaching Based on Anthroposophy
CW 304a	Anthroposophical Knowledge of the Human Being and Pedagogy
CW 305	The Soul-Spiritual Foundational Forces of the Art of Education. Spiritual Values in Education and Social Life
CW 306	Pedagogical Praxis from the Viewpoint of a Spiritual-Scientific Knowledge of the Human Being. The Education of the Child and Young Human Beings
CW 307	The Spiritual Life of the Present and Education
CW 308	The Method of Teaching and the Life-Requirements for Teaching
CW 309	Anthroposophical Pedagogy and Its Prerequisites
CW 310	The Pedagogical Value of a Knowledge of the Human Being and the Cultural Value of Pedagogy
CW 311	The Art of Education from an Understanding of the Being of Humanity
CW 312	Spiritual Science and Medicine
CW 313	Spiritual-Scientific Viewpoints on Therapy
CW 314	Physiology and Therapy Based on Spiritual Science
CW 315	Curative Eurythmy
CW 316	Meditative Observations and Instructions for a Deepening of the Art of Healing
CW 317	The Curative Education Course

CW 318	The Working Together of Doctors and Pastors
CW 319	Anthroposophical Knowledge of the Human Being and Medicine
CW 320	Spiritual-Scientific Impulses for the Development of Physics 1: The First Natural-Scientific Course: Light, Colour, Tone, Mass, Electricity, Magnetism
CW 321	Spiritual-Scientific Impulses for the Development of Physics 2: The Second Natural-Scientific Course: Warmth at the Border of Positive and Negative Materiality
CW 322	The Borders of the Knowledge of Nature
CW 323	The Relationship of the various Natural-Scientific Fields to Astronomy
CW 324	Nature Observation, Mathematics, and Scientific Experimentation and Results from the Viewpoint of Anthroposophy
CW 324a	The Fourth Dimension in Mathematics and Reality
CW 325	Natural Science and the World-Historical Development of Humanity since Ancient Times
CW 326	The Moment of the Coming Into Being of Natural Science in World History and Its Development Since Then
CW 327	Spiritual-Scientific Foundations for Success in Farming. The Agricultural Course
CW 328	The Social Question
CW 329	The Liberation of the Human Being as the Foundation for a New Social Form
CW 330	The Renewal of the Social Organism
CW 331	Work-Council and Socialization
CW 332	The Alliance for Threefolding and the Total Reform of Society. The Council on Culture and the Liberation of the Spiritual Life
CW 332a	The Social Future
CW 333	Freedom of Thought and Social Forces
CW 334	From the Unified State to the Threefold Social Organism
CW 335	The Crisis of the Present and the Path to Healthy Thinking
CW 336	The Great Questions of the Times and Anthroposophical Spiritual Knowledge
CW 337a	Social Ideas, Social Reality, Social Practice, Vol. 1: Question-and-Answer Evenings and Study Evenings of the Alliance for the Threefold Social Organism in Stuttgart, 1919–1920
CW 337b	Social Ideas, Social Realities, Social Practice, Vol. 2: Discussion Evenings of the Swiss Alliance for the Threefold Social Organism
CW 338	How Does One Work on Behalf of the Impulse for the Threefold Social Organism?
CW 339	Anthroposophy, Threefold Social Organism, and the Art of Public Speaking
CW 340	The National-Economics Course. The Tasks of a New Science of Economics, Volume 1
CW 341	The National-Economics Seminar. The Tasks of a New Science of Economics, Volume 2

CW 342	Lectures and Courses on Christian Religious Work, Vol. 1: Anthroposophical Foundations for a Renewed Christian Religious Working
CW 343	Lectures and Courses on Christian Religious Work, Vol. 2: Spiritual Knowledge—Religious Feeling—Cultic Doing
CW 344	Lectures and Courses on Christian Religious Work, Vol. 3: Lectures at the Founding of the Christian Community
CW 345	Lectures and Courses on Christian Religious Work, Vol. 4: Concerning the Nature of the Working Word
CW 346	Lectures and Courses on Christian Religious Work, Vol. 5: The Apocalypse and the Work of the Priest
CW 347	The Knowledge of the Nature of the Human Being According to Body, Soul and Spirit. On Earlier Conditions of the Earth
CW 348	On Health and Illness. Foundations of a Spiritual-Scientific Doctrine of the Senses
CW 349	On the Life of the Human Being and of the Earth. On the Nature of Christianity
CW 350	Rhythms in the Cosmos and in the Human Being. How Does One Come To See the Spiritual World?
CW 351	The Human Being and the World. The Influence of the Spirit in Nature. On the Nature of Bees
CW 352	Nature and the Human Being Observed Spiritual-Scientifically
CW 353	The History of Humanity and the World-Views of the Folk Cultures
CW 354	The Creation of the World and the Human Being. Life on Earth and the Influence of the Stars

SIGNIFICANT EVENTS IN THE LIFE OF RUDOLF STEINER

1829: June 23: birth of Johann Steiner (1829–1910)—Rudolf Steiner's father—in Geras, Lower Austria.

1834: May 8: birth of Franciska Blie (1834–1918)—Rudolf Steiner's mother—in Horn, Lower Austria. 'My father and mother were both children of the glorious Lower Austrian forest district north of the Danube.'

1860: May 16: marriage of Johann Steiner and Franciska Blie.

1861: February 25: birth of *Rudolf Joseph Lorenz Steiner* in Kraljevec, Croatia, near the border with Hungary, where Johann Steiner works as a telegrapher for the South Austria Railroad. Rudolf Steiner is baptized two days later, February 27, the date usually given as his birthday.

1862: Summer: the family moves to Mödling, Lower Austria.

1863: The family moves to Pottschach, Lower Austria, near the Styrian border, where Johann Steiner becomes stationmaster. 'The view stretched to the mountains ... majestic peaks in the distance and the sweet charm of nature in the immediate surroundings.'

1864: November 15: birth of Rudolf Steiner's sister, Leopoldine (d. November 1, 1927). She will become a seamstress and live with her parents for the rest of her life.

1866: July 28: birth of Rudolf Steiner's deaf-mute brother, Gustav (d. May 1, 1941).

1867: Rudolf Steiner enters the village school. Following a disagreement between his father and the schoolmaster, whose wife falsely accused the boy of causing a commotion, Rudolf Steiner is taken out of school and taught at home.

1868: A critical experience. Unknown to the family, an aunt dies in a distant town. Sitting in the station waiting room, Rudolf Steiner sees her 'form,' which speaks to him, asking for help. 'Beginning with this experience, a new soul life began in the boy, one in which not only the outer trees and mountains spoke to him, but also the worlds that lay behind them. From this moment on, the boy began to live with the spirits of nature ...'

1869: The family moves to the peaceful, rural village of Neudorfl, near Wiener-Neustadt in present-day Austria. Rudolf Steiner attends the village school. Because of the 'unorthodoxy' of his writing and spelling, he has to do 'extra lessons.'

1870: Through a book lent to him by his tutor, he discovers geometry: 'To grasp something purely in the spirit brought me inner happiness. I know that I first learned happiness through geometry.' The same tutor allows him to draw, while other students still struggle with their reading and writing. 'An artistic element' thus enters his education.

1871: Though his parents are not religious, Rudolf Steiner becomes a 'church child,' a favourite of the priest, who was 'an exceptional character.' 'Up to the age of ten or eleven, among those I came to know, he was far and away the most significant.' Among other things, he introduces Steiner to Copernican, heliocentric cosmology. As an altar boy, Rudolf Steiner serves at Masses, funerals, and Corpus Christi processions. At year's end, after an incident in which he escapes a thrashing, his father forbids him to go to church.

1872: Rudolf Steiner transfers to grammar school in Wiener-Neustadt, a five-mile walk from home, which must be done in all weathers.

1873–75: Through his teachers and on his own, Rudolf Steiner has many wonderful experiences with science and mathematics. Outside school, he teaches himself analytic geometry, trigonometry, differential equations, and calculus.

1876: Rudolf Steiner begins tutoring other students. He learns bookbinding from his father. He also teaches himself stenography.

1877: Rudolf Steiner discovers Kant's *Critique of Pure Reason*, which he reads and rereads. He also discovers and reads von Rotteck's *World History*.

1878: He studies extensively in contemporary psychology and philosophy.

1879: Rudolf Steiner graduates from high school with honours. His father is transferred to Inzersdorf, near Vienna. He uses his first visit to Vienna 'to purchase a great number of philosophy books'—Kant, Fichte, Schelling, and Hegel, as well as numerous histories of philosophy. His aim: to find a path from the 'I' to nature.

October 1879–1883: Rudolf Steiner attends the Technical College in Vienna—to study mathematics, chemistry, physics, mineralogy, botany, zoology, biology, geology, and mechanics—with a scholarship. He also attends lectures in history and literature, while avidly reading philosophy on his own. His two favourite professors are Karl Julius Schröer (German language and literature) and Edmund Reitlinger (physics). He also audits lectures by Robert Zimmerman on aesthetics and Franz Brentano on philosophy. During this year he begins his friendship with Moritz Zitter (1861–1921), who will help support him financially when he is in Berlin.

1880: Rudolf Steiner attends lectures on Schiller and Goethe by Karl Julius Schröer, who becomes his mentor. Also 'through a remarkable combination of circumstances,' he meets Felix Koguzki, a 'herb gatherer' and healer, who could 'see deeply into the secrets of nature.' Rudolf Steiner will meet and study with this 'emissary of the Master' throughout his time in Vienna.

1881: January: '... I didn't sleep a wink. I was busy with philosophical problems until about 12:30 a.m. Then, finally, I threw myself down on my couch. All my striving during the previous year had been to research whether the following statement by Schelling was true or not: *Within everyone dwells a secret, marvelous capacity to draw back from the stream of time—out of the self clothed in all that comes to us from outside—into our innermost being and there, in the immutable form of the Eternal, to look into ourselves*. I believe, and I am still quite certain of it, that I discovered this capacity in myself; I had long had an inkling of it. Now the whole of idealist philosophy stood before me in modified form. What's a sleepless night compared to that!'

Rudolf Steiner begins communicating with leading thinkers of the day, who send him books in return, which he reads eagerly.

July: 'I am not one of those who dives into the day like an animal in human form. I pursue a quite specific goal, an idealistic aim—knowledge of the truth! This cannot be done offhandedly. It requires the greatest striving in the world, free of all egotism, and equally of all resignation.'

August: Steiner puts down on paper for the first time thoughts for a 'Philosophy of Freedom.' 'The striving for the absolute: this human yearning is freedom.' He also seeks to outline a 'peasant philosophy,' describing what the worldview of a 'peasant'—one who lives close to the earth and the old ways—really is.

1881–1882: Felix Koguzki, the herb gatherer, reveals himself to be the envoy of another, higher initiatory personality, who instructs Rudolf Steiner to penetrate Fichte's philosophy and to master modern scientific thinking as a preparation for right entry into the spirit. This 'Master' also teaches him the double (evolutionary and involutionary) nature of time.

1882: Through the offices of Karl Julius Schröer, Rudolf Steiner is asked by Joseph Kurschner to edit Goethe's scientific works for the *Deutschen National-Literatur* edition. He writes 'A Possible Critique of Atomistic Concepts' and sends it to Friedrich Theodore Vischer.

1883: Rudolf Steiner completes his college studies and begins work on the Goethe project.

1884: First volume of Goethe's *Scientific Writings* (CW 1) appears (March). He lectures on Goethe and Lessing, and Goethe's approach to science. In July, he enters the household of Ladislaus and Pauline Specht as tutor to the four Specht boys. He will live there until 1890. At this time, he meets Josef Breuer (1842–1925), the co-author with Sigmund Freud of *Studies in Hysteria*, who is the Specht family doctor.

1885: While continuing to edit Goethe's writings, Rudolf Steiner reads deeply in contemporary philosophy (Edouard von Hartmann, Johannes Volkelt, and Richard Wahle, among others).

1886: May: Rudolf Steiner sends Kurschner the manuscript of *Outlines of Goethe's Theory of Knowledge* (CW 2), which appears in October, and which he sends out widely. He also meets the poet Marie Eugenie Delle Grazie and writes 'Nature and Our Ideals' for her. He attends her salon, where he meets many priests, theologians, and philosophers, who will become his friends. Meanwhile, the director of the Goethe Archive in Weimar requests his collaboration with the *Sophien* edition of Goethe's works, particularly the writings on colour.

1887: At the beginning of the year, Rudolf Steiner is very sick. As the year progresses and his health improves, he becomes increasingly 'a man of letters,' lecturing, writing essays, and taking part in Austrian cultural life. In August–September, the second volume of Goethe's *Scientific Writings* appears.

1888: January–July: Rudolf Steiner assumes editorship of the 'German Weekly' (*Deutsche Wochenschrift*). He begins lecturing more intensively, giving, for example, a lecture titled 'Goethe as Father of a New Aesthetics.' He meets and becomes soul friends with Friedrich Eckstein (1861–1939), a vegetarian, philosopher of symbolism, alchemist, and musician, who will introduce him to various spiritual currents (including Theosophy) and with whom he will meditate and interpret esoteric and alchemical texts.

1889: Rudolf Steiner first reads Nietzsche (*Beyond Good and Evil*). He encounters Theosophy again and learns of Madame Blavatsky in the Theosophical circle around Marie Lang (1858–1934). Here he also meets well-known figures of Austrian life, as well as esoteric figures like the occultist Franz Hartman and Karl Leinigen-Billigen (translator of C.G. Harrison's *The Transcendental Universe*). During this period, Steiner first reads A.P. Sinnett's *Esoteric Buddhism* and Mabel Collins's *Light on the Path*. He also begins travelling, visiting Budapest, Weimar, and Berlin (where he meets philosopher Edouard von Hartmann).

1890: Rudolf Steiner finishes volume 3 of Goethe's scientific writings. He begins his doctoral dissertation, which will become *Truth and Science* (CW 3). He also meets the poet and feminist Rosa Mayreder (1858–1938), with whom he can exchange his most intimate thoughts. In September, Rudolf Steiner moves to Weimar to work in the Goethe-Schiller Archive.

1891: Volume 3 of the Kurschner edition of Goethe appears. Meanwhile, Rudolf Steiner edits Goethe's studies in mineralogy and scientific writings for the *Sophien* edition. He meets Ludwig Laistner of the Cotta Publishing Company, who asks for a book on the basic question of metaphysics. From this will result, ultimately, *The Philosophy of Freedom* (CW 4), which will be published not by Cotta but by Emil Felber. In October, Rudolf Steiner takes the oral exam for a doctorate in philosophy, mathematics, and mechanics at Rostock University, receiving his doctorate on the twenty-sixth. In November, he gives his first lecture on Goethe's 'Fairy Tale' in Vienna.

1892: Rudolf Steiner continues work at the Goethe-Schiller Archive and on his *Philosophy of Freedom*. *Truth and Science*, his doctoral dissertation, is published. Steiner undertakes to write introductions to books on Schopenhauer and Jean Paul for Cotta. At year's end, he finds lodging with Anna Eunike, née Schulz (1853–1911), a widow with four daughters and a son. He also develops a friendship with Otto Erich Hartleben (1864–1905) with whom he shares literary interests.

1893: Rudolf Steiner begins his habit of producing many reviews and articles. In March, he gives a lecture titled 'Hypnotism, with Reference to Spiritism.' In September, volume 4 of the Kurschner edition is completed. In November, *The Philosophy of Freedom* appears. This year, too, he meets John Henry Mackay (1864–1933), the anarchist, and Max Stirner, a scholar and biographer.

1894: Rudolf Steiner meets Elisabeth Förster Nietzsche, the philosopher's sister, and begins to read Nietzsche in earnest, beginning with the as yet unpublished *Antichrist*. He also meets Ernst Haeckel (1834–1919). In the fall, he begins to write *Nietzsche, A Fighter against His Time* (CW 5).

1895: May, *Nietzsche, A Fighter against His Time* appears.

1896: January 22: Rudolf Steiner sees Friedrich Nietzsche for the first and only time. Moves between the Nietzsche and the Goethe-Schiller Archives, where he completes his work before year's end. He falls out with Elisabeth Förster Nietzsche, thus ending his association with the Nietzsche Archive.

1897: Rudolf Steiner finishes the manuscript of *Goethe's Worldview* (CW 6). He moves to Berlin with Anna Eunike and begins editorship of the *Magazin fur Literatur*. From now on, Steiner will write countless reviews, literary and philosophical articles, and so on. He begins lecturing at the 'Free Literary Society.' In September, he attends the Zionist Congress in Basel. He sides with Dreyfus in the Dreyfus affair.

1898: Rudolf Steiner is very active as an editor in the political, artistic, and theatrical life of Berlin. He becomes friendly with John Henry Mackay and poet Ludwig Jacobowski (1868–1900). He joins Jacobowski's circle of writers, artists, and scientists—'The Coming Ones' (*Die Kommenden*)—and contributes lectures to the group until 1903. He also lectures at the 'League for College Pedagogy.' He writes an article for Goethe's sesquicentennial, 'Goethe's Secret Revelation,' on the 'Fairy Tale of the Green Snake and the Beautiful Lily.'

1898–99: 'This was a trying time for my soul as I looked at Christianity. . . . I was able to progress only by contemplating, by means of spiritual perception, the evolution of Christianity. . . . Conscious knowledge of real Christianity began to dawn in me around the turn of the century. This seed continued to develop. My soul trial occurred shortly before the beginning of the twentieth century. It was decisive for my soul's development that I stood spiritually before the Mystery of Golgotha in a deep and solemn celebration of knowledge.'

1899: Rudolf Steiner begins teaching and giving lectures and lecture cycles at the Workers' College, founded by Wilhelm Liebknecht (1826–1900). He will continue to do so until 1904. Writes: *Literature and Spiritual Life in the Nineteenth Century; Individualism in Philosophy*; *Haeckel and His Opponents; Poetry in the Present;* and begins what will become (fifteen years later) *The Riddles of Philosophy* (CW 18). He also meets many artists and writers, including Käthe Kollwitz, Stefan Zweig, and Rainer Maria Rilke. On October 31, he marries Anna Eunike.

1900: 'I thought that the turn of the century must bring humanity a new light. It seemed to me that the separation of human thinking and willing from the spirit had peaked. A turn or reversal of direction in human evolution seemed to me a necessity.' Rudolf Steiner finishes *World and Life Views in the Nineteenth Century* (the second part of what will become *The Riddles of Philosophy*) and dedicates it to Ernst Haeckel. It is published in March. He continues lecturing at *Die Kommenden*, whose leadership he assumes after the death of Jacobowski. Also, he gives the Gutenberg Jubilee lecture before 7,000 typesetters and printers. In September, Rudolf Steiner is invited by Count and Countess Brockdorff to lecture in the Theosophical Library. His first lecture is on Nietzsche. His second lecture is titled 'Goethe's Secret Revelation.' October 6, he begins a lecture cycle on the mystics that will become *Mystics after Modernism* (CW 7). November-December: 'Marie von Sivers appears in the audience....' Also in November, Steiner gives his first lecture at the Giordano Bruno Bund (where he will continue to lecture until May, 1905). He speaks on Bruno and modern Rome, focusing on the importance of the philosophy of Thomas Aquinas as monism.

1901: In continual financial straits, Rudolf Steiner's early friends Moritz Zitter and Rosa Mayreder help support him. In October, he begins the lecture cycle *Christianity as Mystical Fact* (CW 8) at the Theosophical Library. In November, he gives his first 'Theosophical lecture' on Goethe's 'Fairy Tale' in Hamburg at the invitation of Wilhelm Hubbe-Schleiden. He also attends a gathering to celebrate the founding of the Theosophical Society at Count and Countess Brockdorff's. He gives a lecture cycle, 'From Buddha to Christ,' for the circle of the *Kommenden*. November 17, Marie von Sivers asks Rudolf Steiner if Theosophy needs a Western-Christian spiritual movement (to complement Theosophy's Eastern emphasis). 'The question was posed. Now, following spiritual laws, I could begin to give an answer....' In December, Rudolf Steiner writes his first article for a Theosophical publication. At year's end, the Brockdorffs and possibly Wilhelm Hubbe-Schleiden ask Rudolf Steiner to join the Theosophical Society and undertake the leadership of the German section. Rudolf Steiner agrees, on the condition that Marie von Sivers (then in Italy) work with him.

1902: Beginning in January, Rudolf Steiner attends the opening of the Workers' School in Spandau with Rosa Luxemberg (1870–1919). January 17, Rudolf Steiner joins the Theosophical Society. In April, he is asked to become general secretary of the German Section of the Theosophical Society, and works on preparations for its founding. In July, he visits London for a Theosophical congress. He meets Bertram Keightly, G.R.S. Mead, A.P. Sinnett, and Annie Besant, among others. In September, *Christianity as Mystical Fact* appears. In October, Rudolf Steiner gives his first public lecture on Theosophy ('Monism and Theosophy') to about three hundred people at the Giordano Bruno Bund. On October 19–21, the German Section of the Theosophical Society has its first meeting; Rudolf Steiner is the general secretary, and Annie Besant attends. Steiner lectures on practical karma studies. On October 23, Annie Besant inducts Rudolf Steiner into the Esoteric School of the Theosophical Society. On October 25, Steiner begins a weekly series of lectures: 'The Field of Theosophy.' During this year, Rudolf Steiner also first meets Ita Wegman (1876–1943), who will become his close collaborator in his final years.

1903: Rudolf Steiner holds about 300 lectures and seminars. In May, the first issue of the periodical *Luzifer* appears. In June, Rudolf Steiner visits

London for the first meeting of the Federation of the European Sections of the Theosophical Society, where he meets Colonel Olcott. He begins to write *Theosophy* (CW 9).

1904: Rudolf Steiner continues lecturing at the Workers' College and elsewhere (about 90 lectures), while lecturing intensively all over Germany among Theosophists (about 140 lectures). In February, he meets Carl Unger (1878–1929), who will become a member of the board of the Anthroposophical Society (1913). In March, he meets Michael Bauer (1871–1929), a Christian mystic, who will also be on the board. In May, *Theosophy* appears, with the dedication: 'To the spirit of Giordano Bruno.' Rudolf Steiner and Marie von Sivers visit London for meetings with Annie Besant. June: Rudolf Steiner and Marie von Sivers attend the meeting of the Federation of European Sections of the Theosophical Society in Amsterdam. In July, Steiner begins the articles in *Luzifer-Gnosis* that will become *How to Know Higher Worlds* (CW 10) and *Cosmic Memory* (CW 11). In September, Annie Besant visits Germany. In December, Steiner lectures on Freemasonry. He mentions the High Grade Masonry derived from John Yarker and represented by Theodore Reuss and Karl Kellner as a blank slate 'into which a good image could be placed.'

1905: This year, Steiner ends his non-Theosophical lecturing activity. Supported by Marie von Sivers, his Theosophical lecturing—both in public and in the Theosophical Society—increases significantly: 'The German Theosophical Movement is of exceptional importance.' Steiner recommends reading, among others, Fichte, Jacob Boehme, and Angelus Silesius. He begins to introduce Christian themes into Theosophy. He also begins to work with doctors (Felix Peipers and Ludwig Noll). In July, he is in London for the Federation of European Sections, where he attends a lecture by Annie Besant: 'I have seldom seen Mrs. Besant speak in so inward and heartfelt a manner....' 'Through Mrs. Besant I have found the way to H.P. Blavatsky.' September to October, he gives a course of thirty-one lectures for a small group of esoteric students. In October, the annual meeting of the German Section of the Theosophical Society, which still remains very small, takes place. Rudolf Steiner reports membership has risen from 121 to 377 members. In November, seeking to establish esoteric 'continuity,' Rudolf Steiner and Marie von Sivers participate in a 'Memphis-Misraim' Masonic ceremony. They pay forty-five marks for membership. 'Yesterday, you saw how little remains of former esoteric institutions.' 'We are dealing only with a "framework"... for the present, nothing lies behind it. The occult powers have completely withdrawn.'

1906: Expansion of Theosophical work. Rudolf Steiner gives about 245 lectures, only 44 of which take place in Berlin. Cycles are given in Paris, Leipzig, Stuttgart, and Munich. Esoteric work also intensifies. Rudolf Steiner begins writing *An Outline of Esoteric Science* (CW 13). In January, Rudolf Steiner receives permission (a patent) from the Great Orient of the Scottish A & A Thirty-Three Degree Rite of the Order of the Ancient

Freemasons of the Memphis-Misraim Rite to direct a chapter under the name 'Mystica Aeterna.' This will become the 'Cognitive-Ritual Section' (also called 'Misraim Service') of the Esoteric School. (See: *Freemasonry and Ritual Work: The Misraim Service*, CW 265). During this time, Steiner also meets Albert Schweitzer. In May, he is in Paris, where he visits Edouard Schuré. Many Russians attend his lectures (including Konstantin Balmont, Dimitri Mereszkovski, Zinaida Hippius, and Maximilian Woloshin). He attends the General Meeting of the European Federation of the Theosophical Society, at which Col. Olcott is present for the last time. He spends the year's end in Venice and Rome, where he writes and works on his translation of H.P. Blavatsky's *Key to Theosophy*.

1907: Further expansion of the German Theosophical Movement according to the Rosicrucian directive to 'introduce spirit into the world'—in education, in social questions, in art, and in science. In February, Col. Olcott dies in Adyar. Before he dies, Olcott indicates that 'the Masters' wish Annie Besant to succeed him: much politicking ensues. Rudolf Steiner supports Besant's candidacy. April-May: preparations for the Congress of the Federation of European Sections of the Theosophical Society—the great, watershed Whitsun 'Munich Congress,' attended by Annie Besant and others. Steiner decides to separate Eastern and Western (Christian-Rosicrucian) esoteric schools. He takes his esoteric school out of the Theosophical Society (Besant and Rudolf Steiner are 'in harmony' on this). Steiner makes his first lecture tours to Austria and Hungary. That summer, he is in Italy. In September, he visits Edouard Schuré, who will write the introduction to the French edition of *Christianity as Mystical Fact* in Barr, Alsace. Rudolf Steiner writes the autobiographical statement known as the 'Barr Document.' In *Luzifer-Gnosis*, 'The Education of the Child' appears.

1908: The movement grows (membership: 1,150). Lecturing expands. Steiner makes his first extended lecture tour to Holland and Scandinavia, as well as visits to Naples and Sicily. Themes: St. John's Gospel, the Apocalypse, Egypt, science, philosophy, and logic. *Luzifer-Gnosis* ceases publication. In Berlin, Marie von Sivers (with Johanna Mücke (1864–1949) forms the *Philosophisch-Theosophisch* (after 1915 *Philosophisch-Anthroposophisch*) *Verlag* to publish Steiner's work. Steiner gives lecture cycles titled *The Gospel of St. John* (CW 103) and *The Apocalypse* (104).

1909: *An Outline of Esoteric Science* appears. Lecturing and travel continues. Rudolf Steiner's spiritual research expands to include the polarity of Lucifer and Ahriman; the work of great individualities in history; the Maitreya Buddha and the Bodhisattvas; spiritual economy (CW 109); the work of the spiritual hierarchies in heaven and on earth (CW 110). He also deepens and intensifies his research into the Gospels, giving lectures on the Gospel of St. Luke (CW 114) with the first mention of two Jesus children. Meets and becomes friends with Christian Morgenstern (1871–1914). In April, he lays the foundation stone for the Malsch model—the building that will lead to the first Goetheanum. In May, the International Congress of the Federation of European Sections of the

Theosophical Society takes place in Budapest. Rudolf Steiner receives the Subba Row medal for *How to Know Higher Worlds*. During this time, Charles W. Leadbeater discovers Jiddu Krishnamurti (1895–1986) and proclaims him the future 'world teacher,' the bearer of the Maitreya Buddha and the 'reappearing Christ.' In October, Steiner delivers seminal lectures on 'anthroposophy,' which he will try, unsuccessfully, to rework over the next years into the unfinished work, *Anthroposophy (A Fragment)* (CW 45).

1910: New themes: *The Reappearance of Christ in the Etheric* (CW 118); *The Fifth Gospel; The Mission of Folk Souls* (CW 121); *Occult History* (CW 126); the evolving development of etheric cognitive capacities. Rudolf Steiner continues his Gospel research with *The Gospel of St. Matthew* (CW 123). In January, his father dies. In April, he takes a month-long trip to Italy, including Rome, Monte Cassino, and Sicily. He also visits Scandinavia again. July–August, he writes the first mystery drama, *The Portal of Initiation* (CW 14). In November, he gives 'psychosophy' lectures. In December, he submits 'On the Psychological Foundations and Epistemological Framework of Theosophy' to the International Philosophical Congress in Bologna.

1911: The crisis in the Theosophical Society deepens. In January, 'The Order of the Rising Sun,' which will soon become 'The Order of the Star in the East,' is founded for the coming world teacher, Krishnamurti. At the same time, Marie von Sivers, Rudolf Steiner's co-worker, falls ill. Fewer lectures are given, but important new ground is broken. In Prague, in March, Steiner meets Franz Kafka (1883–1924) and Hugo Bergmann (1883-1975). In April, he delivers his paper to the Philosophical Congress. He writes the second mystery drama, *The Soul's Probation* (CW 14). Also, while Marie von Sivers is convalescing, Rudolf Steiner begins work on *Calendar 1912/1913*, which will contain the 'Calendar of the Soul' meditations. On March 19, Anna (Eunike) Steiner dies. In September, Rudolf Steiner visits Einsiedeln, birthplace of Paracelsus. In December, Friedrich Rittelmeyer, future founder of the Christian Community, meets Rudolf Steiner. The *Johannes-Bauverein*, the 'building committee,' which would lead to the first Goetheanum (first planned for Munich), is also founded, and a preliminary committee for the founding of an independent association is created that, in the following year, will become the Anthroposophical Society. Important lecture cycles include *Occult Physiology* (CW 128); *Wonders of the World* (CW 129); *From Jesus to Christ* (CW 131). Other themes: esoteric Christianity; Christian Rosenkreutz; the spiritual guidance of humanity; the sense world and the world of the spirit.

1912: Despite the ongoing, now increasing crisis in the Theosophical Society, much is accomplished: *Calendar 1912/1913* is published; eurythmy is created; both the third mystery drama, *The Guardian of the Threshold* (CW 14) and *A Way of Self-Knowledge* (CW 16) are written. New (or renewed) themes included life between death and rebirth and karma and reincarnation. Other lecture cycles: *Spiritual Beings in the Heavenly Bodies and in the Kingdoms of Nature* (CW 136); *The Human Being in the Light of Occultism, Theosophy, and Philosophy* (CW 137); *The Gospel of St. Mark* (CW 139); and *The Bhagavad Gita and the Epistles of Paul* (CW 142). On May 8, Rudolf Steiner celebrates White Lotus Day, H.P. Blavatsky's death day, which he had faithfully observed for the past decade, for the last time. In August, Rudolf Steiner suggests the 'independent association' be called the 'Anthroposophical Society.' In September, the first eurythmy course takes place. In October, Rudolf Steiner declines recognition of a Theosophical Society lodge dedicated to the Star of the East and decides to expel all Theosophical Society members belonging to the order. Also, with Marie von Sivers, he first visits Dornach, near Basel, Switzerland, and they stand on the hill where the Goetheanum will be built. In November, a Theosophical Society lodge is opened by direct mandate from Adyar (Annie Besant). In December, a meeting of the German section occurs at which it is decided that belonging to the Order of the Star of the East is incompatible with membership in the Theosophical Society. December 28: informal founding of the Anthroposophical Society in Berlin.

1913: Expulsion of the German section from the Theosophical Society. February 2–3: Foundation meeting of the Anthroposophical Society. Board members include: Marie von Sivers, Michael Bauer, and Carl Unger. September 20: Laying of the foundation stone for the *Johannes Bau* (Goetheanum) in Dornach. Building begins immediately. The third mystery drama, *The Soul's Awakening* (CW 14), is completed. Also: *The Threshold of the Spiritual World* (CW 147). Lecture cycles include: *The Bhagavad Gita and the Epistles of Paul* and *The Esoteric Meaning of the Bhagavad Gita* (CW 146), which the Russian philosopher Nikolai Berdyaev attends; *The Mysteries of the East and of Christianity* (CW 144); *The Effects of Esoteric Development* (CW 145); and *The Fifth Gospel* (CW 148). In May, Rudolf Steiner is in London and Paris, where anthroposophical work continues.

1914: Building continues on the *Johannes Bau* (Goetheanum) in Dornach, with artists and co-workers from seventeen nations. The general assembly of the Anthroposophical Society takes place. In May, Rudolf Steiner visits Paris, as well as Chartres Cathedral. June 28: assassination in Sarajevo ('Now the catastrophe has happened!'). August 1: War is declared. Rudolf Steiner returns to Germany from Dornach—he will travel back and forth. He writes the last chapter of *The Riddles of Philosophy*. Lecture cycles include: *Human and Cosmic Thought* (CW 151); *Inner Being of Humanity between Death and a New Birth* (CW 153); *Occult Reading and Occult Hearing* (CW 156). December 24: marriage of Rudolf Steiner and Marie von Sivers.

1915: Building continues. Life after death becomes a major theme, also art. Writes: *Thoughts during a Time of War* (CW 24). Lectures include: *The Secret of Death* (CW 159); *The Uniting of Humanity through the Christ Impulse* (CW 165).

1916: Rudolf Steiner begins work with Edith Maryon (1872–1924) on the sculpture 'The Representative of Humanity' ('The Group'—Christ, Lucifer, and Ahriman). He also works with the alchemist Alexander von Bernus on the quarterly *Das Reich*. He writes *The Riddle of Humanity* (CW 20). Lectures include: *Necessity and Freedom in World History and Human Action* (CW 166); *Past and Present in the Human Spirit* (CW 167); *The Karma of Vocation* (CW 172); *The Karma of Untruthfulness* (CW 173).

1917: Russian Revolution. The U.S. enters the war. Building continues. Rudolf Steiner delineates the idea of the 'threefold nature of the human being' (in a public lecture March 15) and the 'threefold nature of the social organism' (hammered out in May-June with the help of Otto von Lerchenfeld and Ludwig Polzer-Hoditz in the form of two documents titled *Memoranda*, which were distributed in high places). August–September: Rudolf Steiner writes *The Riddles of the Soul* (CW 20). Also: commentary on 'The Chemical Wedding of Christian Rosenkreutz' for Alexander Bernus (*Das Reich*). Lectures include: *The Karma of Materialism* (CW 176); *The Spiritual Background of the Outer World: The Fall of the Spirits of Darkness* (CW 177).

1918: March 18: peace treaty of Brest-Litovsk—'Now everything will truly enter chaos! What is needed is cultural renewal.' June: Rudolf Steiner visits Karlstein (Grail) Castle outside Prague. Lecture cycle: *From Symptom to Reality in Modern History* (CW 185). In mid-November, Emil Molt, of the Waldorf-Astoria Cigarette Company, has the idea of founding a school for his workers' children.

1919: Focus on the threefold social organism: tireless travel, countless lectures, meetings, and publications. At the same time, a new public stage of Anthroposophy emerges as cultural renewal begins. The coming years will see initiatives in pedagogy, medicine, pharmacology, and agriculture. January 27: threefold meeting: ' We must first of all, with the money we have, found free schools that can bring people what they need.' February: first public eurythmy performance in Zurich. Also: 'Appeal to the German People' (CW 24), circulated March 6 as a newspaper insert. In April, *Towards Social Renewal* (CW 23) appears—'perhaps the most widely read of all books on politics appearing since the war.' Rudolf Steiner is asked to undertake the 'direction and leadership' of the school founded by the Waldorf-Astoria Company. Rudolf Steiner begins to talk about the 'renewal' of education. May 30: a building is selected and purchased for the future Waldorf School. August–September, Rudolf Steiner gives a lecture course for Waldorf teachers, *The Foundations of Human Experience (Study of Man)* (CW 293). September 7: Opening of the first Waldorf School. December (into January): first science course, the *Light Course* (CW 320).

1920: The Waldorf School flourishes. New threefold initiatives. Founding of limited companies *Der Kommende Tag* and *Futurum A.G.* to infuse spiritual values into the economic realm. Rudolf Steiner also focuses on the sciences. Lectures: *Introducing Anthroposophical Medicine* (CW 312); *The Warmth Course* (CW 321); *The Boundaries of Natural Science* (CW 322); *The Redemption of Thinking* (CW 74). February: Johannes Werner

Klein—later a co-founder of the Christian Community—asks Rudolf Steiner about the possibility of a 'religious renewal,' a 'Johannine church.' In March, Rudolf Steiner gives the first course for doctors and medical students. In April, a divinity student asks Rudolf Steiner a second time about the possibility of religious renewal. September 27–October 16: anthroposophical 'university course.' December: lectures titled *The Search for the New Isis* (CW 202).

1921: Rudolf Steiner continues his intensive work on cultural renewal, including the uphill battle for the threefold social order. 'University' arts, scientific, theological, and medical courses include: *The Astronomy Course* (CW 323); *Observation, Mathematics, and Scientific Experiment* (CW 324); the *Second Medical Course* (CW 313); *Colour*. In June and September-October, Rudolf Steiner also gives the first two 'priests' courses' (CW 342 and 343). The 'youth movement' gains momentum. Magazines are founded: *Die Drei* (January), and—under the editorship of Albert Steffen (1884–1963)—the weekly, *Das Goetheanum* (August). In February–March, Rudolf Steiner takes his first trip outside Germany since the war (Holland). On April 7, Steiner receives a letter regarding 'religious renewal,' and May 22–23, he agrees to address the question in a practical way. In June, the Klinical-Therapeutic Institute opens in Arlesheim under the direction of Dr. Ita Wegman. In August, the Chemical-Pharmaceutical Laboratory opens in Arlesheim (Oskar Schmiedel and Ita Wegman are directors). The Clinical Therapeutic Institute is inaugurated in Stuttgart (Dr. Ludwig Noll is director); also the Research Laboratory in Dornach (Ehrenfried Pfeiffer and Gunther Wachsmuth are directors). In November–December, Rudolf Steiner visits Norway.

1922: The first half of the year involves very active public lecturing (thousands attend); in the second half, Rudolf Steiner begins to withdraw and turn toward the Society—'The Society is asleep.' It is 'too weak' to do what is asked of it. The businesses—*Der Kommende Tag* and *Futurum A.G.*—fail. In January, with the help of an agent, Steiner undertakes a twelve-city German lecture tour, accompanied by eurythmy performances. In two weeks he speaks to more than 2,000 people. In April, he gives a 'university course' in The Hague. He also visits England. In June, he is in Vienna for the East–West Congress. In August–September, he is back in England for the Oxford Conference on Education. Returning to Dornach, he gives the lectures *Philosophy, Cosmology, and Religion* (CW 215), and gives the third priests' course (CW 344). On September 16, The Christian Community is founded. In October–November, Steiner is in Holland and England. He also speaks to the youth: *The Youth Course* (CW 217). In December, Steiner gives lectures titled *The Origins of Natural Science* (CW 326), and *Humanity and the World of Stars: The Spiritual Communion of Humanity* (CW 219). December 31: Fire at the Goetheanum, which is destroyed.

1923: Despite the fire, Rudolf Steiner continues his work unabated. A very hard year. Internal dispersion, dissension, and apathy abound. There is conflict—between old and new visions—within the Society. A wake-up call is needed, and Rudolf Steiner responds with renewed lecturing vitality. His focus: the spiritual context of human life; initiation science; the course of the year; and community building. As a foundation for an artistic school, he creates a series of pastel sketches. Lecture cycles: *The Anthroposophical Movement; Initiation Science* (CW 227) (in England at the Penmaenmawr Summer School); *The Four Seasons and the Archangels* (CW 229); *Harmony of the Creative Word* (CW 230); *The Supersensible Human* (CW 231), given in Holland for the founding of the Dutch society. On November 10, in response to the failed Hitler-Ludendorff putsch in Munich, Steiner closes his Berlin residence and moves the *Philosophisch-Anthroposophisch Verlag* (Press) to Dornach. On December 9, Steiner begins the serialization of his *Autobiography: The Course of My Life* (CW 28) in *Das Goetheanum*. It will continue to appear weekly, without a break, until his death. Late December–early January: Rudolf Steiner re-founds the Anthroposophical Society (about 12,000 members internationally) and takes over its leadership. The new board members are: Marie Steiner, Ita Wegman, Albert Steffen, Elizabeth Vreede, and Guenther Wachsmuth. (See *The Christmas Meeting for the Founding of the General Anthroposophical Society*, CW 260). Accompanying lectures: *Mystery Knowledge and Mystery Centres* (CW 232); *World History in the Light of Anthroposophy* (CW 233). December 25: the Foundation Stone is laid (in the hearts of members) in the form of the 'Foundation Stone Meditation.'

1924: January 1: having founded the Anthroposophical Society and taken over its leadership, Rudolf Steiner has the task of 'reforming' it. The process begins with a weekly newssheet ('What's Happening in the Anthroposophical Society') in which Rudolf Steiner's 'Letters to Members' and 'Anthroposophical Leading Thoughts' appear (CW 26). The next step is the creation of a new esoteric class, the 'first class' of the 'University of Spiritual Science' (which was to have been followed, had Rudolf Steiner lived longer, by two more advanced classes). Then comes a new language for Anthroposophy—practical, phenomenological, and direct; and Rudolf Steiner creates the model for the second Goetheanum. He begins the series of extensive 'karma' lectures (CW 235–40); and finally, responding to needs, he creates two new initiatives: biodynamic agriculture and curative education. After the middle of the year, rumours begin to circulate regarding Steiner's health. Lectures: January–February, *Anthroposophy* (CW 234); February: *Tone Eurythmy* (CW 278); June: *The Agriculture Course* (CW 327); June–July: *Speech Eurythmy* (CW 279); *Curative Education* (CW 317); August: (England, 'Second International Summer School'), *Initiation Consciousness: True and False Paths in Spiritual Investigation* (CW 243); September: *Pastoral Medicine* (CW 318). On September 26, for the first time, Rudolf Steiner cancels a lecture. On September 28, he gives his last lecture. On September 29, he withdraws to his studio in the carpenter's shop; now he is definitively ill. Cared for by Ita Wegman, he continues working, however, and writing the weekly installments of his *Autobiography* and *Letters to the Members/Leading Thoughts* (CW 26).

1925: Rudolf Steiner, while continuing to work, continues to weaken. He finishes *Extending Practical Medicine* (CW 27) with Ita Wegman.
On March 30, around ten in the morning, Rudolf Steiner dies.

INDEX

A NOTE FROM RUDOLF STEINER PRESS

We are an independent publisher and registered charity (non-profit organisation) dedicated to making available the work of Rudolf Steiner in English translation. We care a great deal about the content of our books and have hundreds of titles available – as printed books, ebooks and in audio formats.

As a publisher devoted to anthroposophy...

- We continually commission translations of previously unpublished works by Rudolf Steiner and invest in re-translating, editing and improving our editions.
- We are committed to making anthroposophy available to all by publishing introductory books as well as contemporary research.
- Our new print editions and ebooks are carefully checked and proofread for accuracy, and converted into all formats for all platforms.
- Our translations are officially authorised by Rudolf Steiner's estate in Dornach, Switzerland, to whom we pay royalties on sales, thus assisting their critical work.

So, look out for Rudolf Steiner Press as a mark of quality and support us today by buying our books, or contact us should you wish to sponsor specific titles or to support the charity with a gift or legacy.